What People...
The Way Out . . .

"*The Way Out* is a practical and refreshingly honest roadmap for gay men whose journey just begins with 'coming out.' Christopher Nutter's own self-exploration identifies real challenges for gay men, and gives insights and tools to help us be our best selves."

Alan Van Capelle
Executive Director, Empire State Pride

"Written with humor, insight, hope and faith, *The Way Out* may prove to be an enduring 'post-gay' survival guide for the twenty-first century gay man."

Jack Drescher, M.D.
Author, *Psychoanalytic Therapy and the Gay Man*

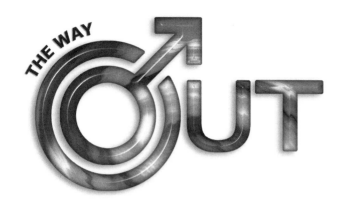

THE WAY OUT

The Gay Man's Guide to Freedom No Matter If You're in Denial, in the Closet, One Foot Out, Just Out or Been Around the Block

CHRISTOPHER LEE NUTTER

Health Communications, Inc.
Deerfield Beach, Florida

www.bcibooks.com

Library of Congress Cataloging-in-Publication Data
is available at the Library of Congress.

Nutter, Christopher Lee.

©2006 Christopher Lee Nutter
ISBN 0-7573-0392-7

Publisher: Health Communications, Inc.
            3201 S.W. 15th Street
            Deerfield Beach, FL 33442-8190

Cover design by Larissa Hise Henoch
Inside book design by Dawn Von Strolley Grove

This book is dedicated to my Mom, Betty, who taught me both about the nature of wisdom and the power of writing.

Contents

Acknowledgments

I would like to thank my agent Robert Guinsler at Sterling Lord Literistic for being as dedicated as he is talented; my editor Amy Hughes for dropping my dream project right in my lap; Sagi Haviv, who designed the symbol on the cover of the book, for sharing his genius and his love so freely; Atila Marquez who took the author photo for being such a brilliant photographer and a good friend.

Alan Van Capelle, Dr. Jack Drescher, and Neil Giuliano for making the time to read this book and so graciously extending their hard won respect to it; Quohnos Mitchell at Tommy Hilfger Europe for dressing me for all of my personal appearances; Steven Ward for styling my hair at the photo shoot.

Kim Weiss and Julie De La Cruz at HCI for being the PR team from heaven; Richard Goldstein who mentored me at the *Village Voice* for telling me that what I had to say and how I said it was valid; my brother Jason and my mom Betty for always supporting me so selflessly and wholeheartedly; every gay man who came before me who fought much

Acknowledgments

worse monsters than I did; every gay activist for making my life as it has been a possibility; and every gay man today who, through their sheer existence, are teaching me how to love.

Introduction: Finding My Way Out

This above all, to thine own self be true.

—William Shakespeare

I have spent my entire life looking for the way out of pain.

However, no matter what form it took—fear, depression, bitterness, anxiety, jealousy, loneliness, addiction, anger, judgment, self-criticism, you name it—and no matter how much it hurt, for most of my life I didn't think of it as pain. Rather I qualified these feelings as symptoms of my imperfection. In other words, I thought the pain was me.

As an adolescent growing up in the suburbs of Birmingham, Alabama, in the '70s and '80s, I was in a lot of pain. But by the time I was sixteen, I was sick enough of being listless and depressed to do something about it. I decided that I wanted to be happy. And I was certain that the way to do this was to correct my imperfections.

The most serious of these imperfections was my homosexuality—it was my fatal flaw, my original sin that I had not chosen to commit. Though by my midteens I had accepted that this condition was never going to change, I could not really accept that I was gay. To me that would have meant accepting that I was a lonely, pitiful and defective human being, that I was not loved by God, that I was *less* than straight men, that the only others like me were shadowy discards from society. Doing that would have meant accepting that I was never going to be happy, so that was out of the question.

My sexual attraction to men, however, was by no means the only imperfection I needed to cloak. Compared to the fabulous *Pretty in Pink* teens I grew up with, I was absolutely riddled with imperfections—I wasn't beautiful; I wasn't rich; I wasn't masculine; I wasn't confident; I wasn't athletic. As I became hyperaware of these inadequacies, too, I slowly became both ashamed and embarrassed to be me.

To remedy this I became devoted to getting gorgeous and becoming popular—in other words, to getting "perfect." And college became the set where I was able to successfully act the role of a privileged pretty boy. Playing this role felt like the very first shot of morphine after a lifetime of debilitating pain, and I often felt high. But whenever the morphine wore off, I would find myself hurtling back into the void, and it was as if I had never left.

Meanwhile, my sexuality was literally in the closet—that's where I kept my gay porn, on a high shelf in a small closet blocked off by a large chair. I even did such a number on myself that, whenever I saw a guy I thought was gay, I would find myself thinking, "Ugh, how horrible that would be." Then I would momentarily move into a kind of twilight zone of awareness of the fact that *I* was this person I pitied. I was in a state of shock over my own being.

Then in 1993 I made a monumental shift in how I experienced my life when I rebelled against the depression that still tormented me and looked inside myself for the first time for its source in the form of my own thoughts. Not only did learning how to fight my thoughts mark the beginning of the end of depression for me, it awoke a nascent awareness of my power to change the reality of my life by looking inward rather than outward. As a result, the way I lived my life began to change.

First I ditched my plans to go to law school and decided instead to follow my lifelong dream to become a writer. Even more significant, for the first time in my life I began to question my belief that I couldn't come out of the closet and be happy. There were few images of gay people in the media then, so it was still a very lonely time to be gay. And I couldn't even say the word "gay" out loud, so I was at a total loss as to how to go about coming out.

Then opportunity struck. One night I read in *Details* magazine that they were starting a new section that readers could submit stories for. And I had a revelation: I would write an essay about life inside the closet and thereby come out in the process. As much as going through with it scared me, and as much as it seemed an impossible long shot that it would be selected, I became aware of a silent, certain knowledge about what to do next: write that essay. And so I did.

Despite my sense of certainty, I was shocked when I got a call from an editor in New York saying they loved the piece and wanted to run it with a picture. At the time I was getting ready to move from Mississippi, where I'd gone to college, to Boston for my first magazine internship. Added to the mix of my new life "up North" and working in publishing would be the fact that I would be Out. Me. Out of the closet. Gay and for everyone else to see. I couldn't even imagine it.

The impact of this article had a tectonic effect on my life, and the result was miraculous. When the issue hit the stands I was, in one swoop, out to the world. And quite unlike my fears of rejection, I actually received a flood of warm congratulations from friends and family. Then the real shock came when dozens of young gay men from all over the country began to write and call looking for guidance. I myself was now a gay image in the media, and a coming out mini-guru. It blew my mind.

Most miraculous of all, though, were my feelings. I was the same person I was the day before, only significantly truer to myself, and it felt amazing. I was, to put it mildly, in a state of bliss, reborn.

The big lesson for me was that it had been *my own ideas* that I had to be a different person from who I truly was in order to be happy that had prevented me from experiencing the bliss of authenticity. Growing up, my mom would regularly quote William Shakespeare: "This above all, to thine own self be true." Finally I understood what she, and Shakespeare, meant.

It wasn't for another year and a half after I'd moved to New York City that I decided to become "gay" in the cultural sense because I was terrified to let go of the "straight" Southern frat boy sensibilities I had cultivated so carefully. The first guy I slept with—a very "straight-acting" guy I met on the subway—only reinforced these notions, for he, too, slept with men but wanted nothing to do with "gay life" because he was a "real man." But when my roommate, Dean, took me out to a legendary club in downtown Manhattan called the Tunnel, and I popped an ecstasy and got a load of gorgeous, glamorous gay men with hot bodies, I changed my tune. I thought, if *this* is what being gay is, I want to be it.

By the time I was twenty-seven I felt I had arrived: I was a bartender at a famous gay bar, scored a gig as a nightlife columnist for a gay magazine, had become a known party boy in both Manhattan and Miami Beach, and laid myself out in a black-and-white spread for a Rizzoli book of homoerotic nudes. And just like in college, I was high as a kite from my successes. But it was an extremely fragile feeling, and all it took was a guy not calling me back to then have to spend weeks getting control of my thoughts again in order to recover from depression. It seemed no matter how "perfect" I got, the void would always get me in the end.

By the time I was twenty-nine, after four jam-packed years mastering gay life, I was spent. As Etta James would sing in the blues bars in Mississippi, the thrill was gone. And what it would take to get the high back—harder drugs, riskier sex, getting supersized by steroids—I wasn't willing to do. I still longed to be happy, but that route looked like an express train to the grave.

So I felt I had no choice but to drop out of the scene. From that point I lived in a state of withdrawal from all the morphine, in the form of attention, I had become addicted to. Looking for some kind of compensatory rush, I found myself compulsively gorging on sexual conquests, and after two years of that I found myself functionally impotent. By that time the emptiness I felt had crept into everything I did. I felt, in a word, bereft.

It began to dawn on me that I knew a lot about being high, but not much about being happy. I needed answers. I needed a way out. But it was not easy to find. Gay culture continued to advertise the dream of gay heaven—that the right boyfriend, the right party, and the right sexual conquest was the answer—but I'd wound up in hell. And well-meaning gay friends and mentors suggested that my real problem was that I was just thinking about it all way, way, way too much.

Of course, the problem wasn't that I was thinking too much. It's that I was seeing more deeply.

Then one day I was sitting out on my stoop on 21st Street in the heart of gay Chelsea brooding over the tremendous sense of loss I was living in when the wordless voice spoke up again, and I knew to get up and go to the bookstore. I marched two avenues over to the Barnes & Noble and walked directly to a book I recognized as the one I needed to read immediately.

It was the Dalai Lama's *Transforming the Mind*. I picked it up and read something that resonated through my being: not only does all suffering emanate from my thoughts, but I have the power to change my thoughts.

And so I got to work. Gay party boy became gay spiritual boy. At first, it was torture. I lived in a virtual isolation tank and became an audience to the movies playing in my head, no matter how painful they were. And with no one to project the movies on and precious little to anesthetize the pain they caused me, I discovered something profound.

I discovered that *I* was the creator of my life, not a victim of it, and I created in two ways—consciously in a state of aware-ness, and unconsciously without awareness.

This helped me discover the true nature of my emotional pain, which I unconsciously created with my own thoughts. Being unaware of this, I believed that the pain came from out-side of me or was an intrinsic part of me. Consciously I could see what I had been doing and with the power this knowledge gave me, I could stop using my own mind against myself, end-ing the need for anesthesia to cover the pain up or internal battles to fight it off. And as I began to heal I discovered that an infinite abundance of happiness existed inside me; all I had to do was to learn how to want it, and how to receive it.

Though I was putting all this newfound insight into practice, for a long time I still felt empty and removed, and in a great deal of conflict. It was as if I had one foot in my old life but the other foot was still hanging in the air.

Then one misty April Sunday evening after about a year and a half of living in limbo like this, the other foot hit. I was walk-ing down 22nd Street between 5th and 6th Avenues when I was suddenly awash in something I can only describe as extreme clarity and awareness. I was then hit by a tidal wave of bliss that was so consuming and brought such tears and convulsions that I could barely walk (though I held it together enough to cross the street to avoid people, who surely would have called 911 had they seen me up close). Though at first I didn't understand what was happening, slowly as I made my way home I realized that I had become *connected* to who I truly am, which is pure consciousness. At that moment I was infused with the very antidote to feeling bereft. That one moment of realization was enough to change me forever.

What I have gone through and continue to go through has been experienced by many people throughout the ages. But what made bringing my own path to light so challenging was the fact that there was almost no mention of gay people or the gay experience in any tradition I explored. This glaring absence is mystifying to me, but there is no need to investigate it. The same truth applies to everyone on Earth, and the same light exists in every person. But gay men, like every other group, have a unique path tailored especially for our growth. This book is intended to help you see how your life as a gay man is, in fact, tailored with perfect precision so that you, too, can discover who you truly are. In that way, as my friend Thomas says, being gay is a gift, and this book is here in part to help you realize it.

Coming out of the closet is usually thought of as the singular answer to the gay "predicament." As transformative as it is, coming out is not enough, for there is now a gay world ready to take over your mind and fill your head with yet another "reality" about who you are. All you have to do these days is become conscious enough to realize you aren't straight, move over into gay society, and then slip right back into unconsciousness by letting gay society tell you who you are and who you should be. It's like waking up from a coma in intensive care only long enough to shuffle over to another unit where the bed is a better fit and the pain medication is more intense and then going right back to sleep. And because of this, like practically every other group on the planet, gay men are having what the philosopher Joseph Campbell called a "schizophrenic crack-up" from aligning ourselves with gay culture's programmatic life rather than listening to our own hearts.

And these days we are being assaulted with programming from every direction. Gay culture itself bombards its denizens with views of ourselves at once outlandishly self-aggrandizing and tragically self-destructive. Mainstream popular culture, once virtually silent about our existence, is now telling us we are genetically programmed to be "fabulous," but please don't have our gay sex or our gay love anywhere in the open. And many of our political and religious leaders are waging what they say they believe is a holy war to keep gay people from receiving any sort of societal or spiritual support and legitimacy.

Living at the center of this tornado, every gay man is left to ask himself, am I the coolest, trendiest, sexiest thing ever, or an illegitimate cancer on society?

Which is it?

The answer is that we are neither. In fact, we are not even gay. We are, like everyone on the planet, spiritual beings on a physical quest to realize our true nature. And the only way to the realization of this truth is through the process of *letting go* of everything you think you know, of every limit you are sure exists, of every fear that has gone unquestioned; for letting go is the only way to make room in your mind for something new. The book *A Course in Miracles* points out that your perception only allows in what it already believes to be true, so if you are not willing to let go of your existing beliefs, you have no chance of seeing that you, too, are the sole creator of your life, and you have more power than you could ever imagine.

Letting go includes letting go of any ideas you might have about what "spirituality" or "consciousness" or "God" or even "gay" means, because they are just symbols on a map, nothing more. Don't get hung up on them. And trust me, this something new that letting go will reveal is utterly miraculous. The point isn't just to accept or reject this, but to test it out to see if it might be true for you too.

As anyone who knows me will tell you, I am not perfect. As Candi Staton sang so poignantly in the old disco classic, "I'm a victim of the very song I sing." However, like many others, I have been given a message that I put into practice every day, and that I am here, now, to pass on. And it is that, indeed, I am perfect. And so are you. We are perfection itself . . . just not yet realized.

♂² Come Out Consciously, and Stay Out Consciously, *Even If You Are Already Out*

The hero gets the adventure he's ready for.

—Joseph Campbell

When I came out at the age of twenty-four, my mom told me that she'd known I was gay since I was a toddler. When I asked her why she had never brought it up, she told me that she had adopted the same policy as a doctor she knew. When he would operate on a tumor, if it was benign, he would volunteer the information as soon as the patient woke up. If it was cancerous, he would wait until the patient asked. Why? Because if they asked, it meant they were ready for the truth. With that in mind, she said she decided that when I was ready to talk about my sexuality, when I was ready for the truth, I would bring it up.

This is the central condition we as gay men find ourselves in—waking up in this life to what is generally considered bad news or even very bad news, and having to decide for ourselves when we're ready for the truth. However, rather than seeing this condition as a misfortune as it is generally thought of, coming out to oneself and to the world is in fact an amazing opportunity for self-realization. It is, in fact, good news.

I'm not trying to pretend that it's "rah-rah" good news like getting a promotion at work or getting bumped up to first class is good news. Rather, it's good news on a much deeper and more meaningful level—the kind of news that leads to the end of the need for "first class" as we know it in its finite and fragile physical form, and the beginning of being able to experience the entire world as first class because everything is divine, and everything is meaningful.

Of course, like all serious challenges, in the heat of things it doesn't feel "good" at all. It feels brutal, terrifying and unfair. (After all, you didn't choose this!) You wake up to your existence living under an assumption of your straightness—living as it were in the Straight Shining City on the Hill—only to slowly discover within yourself that you are an imposter, even to your own family. Most, as I did, peep down over the edge into the darkened valley of the "other" and think, "I don't want to live there. I belong here."

But you know in your heart you don't belong. And knowing that once you announce you are gay a trap door is going to open and down you're gonna slide into the valley of the "other," like Keanu Reeves getting kicked out of the Matrix, is no easy destiny.

Gay men who come out because they decide that their happiness is more important than holding on to their fears find that the valley of "the other" and the Straight Shining City on the Hill no longer exist if we don't believe in them. By being brave enough to cross this mighty chasm between fear and freedom, we empower ourselves to rely on our own awareness to judge what is true and untrue about ourselves, freeing us from the judgments of the world forever, and in the process discovering the awesome power we have to create reality in accordance with our own will. In doing so, we become citizens of the only Shining City on the Hill there is, which is the Kingdom of Heaven within. *That* is the moment that the crisis of being gay in this world transmutes into opportunity for profound realization.

This is the essence of the gift of being gay, for while straight people have it "easier" in the worldly sense—and it is truly a first-class world for straight people—they do not have it easier when it comes to waking up from unconsciousness because they are not challenged in the profound way that gay people are. And that's where it counts. After all, what straight person in the world has ever had to take a giant leap of consciousness just to acknowledge the gender they are sexually attracted to? And can you look around the world today at all the unimaginable suffering of literally billions of straight people and tell me that straight people are happier and more at peace in the midst of their "first-class" existence? It just doesn't work that way because the idea that being straight is better is an illusion.

Being gay is a special gift for men because by coming out we willfully trade in our great place of privilege in the world for a greater sense of our true selves. And even other subjugated groups—women, people of color—usually don't get the particular challenge and opportunity for growth that *choice* offers.

The opportunities lie in which choices you make. However, the infinite number of choices gay men have to make in their lives in the matter of coming out is truly harrowing. To begin to understand the significance of these choices, it is necessary to begin by understanding what being "out" means in the first place.

What Is "Out"?

To define "out," you first have to define what "in" is. After all, "in" creates "out," so you cannot have one without the other.

"In the closet" is a metaphor to describe the choice the vast majority of gay men make at one point or another in their lives to hide their sexual nature. By hiding, you do not change your nature, you only put it out of sight from yourself and from others. It is this positioning that requires that a person "come out" in order to reveal the truth about his sexual nature. And there is nothing at all *wrong* with being in the closet—it's just the best choice a gay person knows how to make at a particular time given the unfavorable conditions of the world in which we live. It is a natural defense mechanism, and I made that decision, too.

"Out of the closet," then, is measured by the degree to which you are no longer "in the closet"—in other words, the degree to which you no longer hide your true sexual nature. Given that this is an exclusively internal process, the first degree of "out" is being out to yourself; in other words, to acknowledge to yourself that you are sexually attracted to men. In this case, you know that you are gay, but you do not share this with anyone because you are afraid of the consequences.

The next degree to being "out" occurs when you are no longer as afraid of the consequences, or when you've decided for yourself that the consequences will be better, or couldn't be worse, than life in the closet. The degree to which you do acknowledge it to others is based entirely on the degree to which you realize the deep truth underneath all the lies about yourself that you absorbed from the world around you—that there is nothing wrong with being gay, and, therefore, there is no reason to hide it. Realizing this can be an incredibly long journey and few gay men ever make it, but when you achieve that level of "outness," then you have transcended the closet altogether—you no longer have to be "out" because no part of you is "in." You simply *are*.

Coming Out 101

When it comes to coming out, there are two essential intents. On the one hand is the intent to do as little self-examination as possible in order to get what your ego—which is to say your identification with the part of you that lives in fear—wants from being out (sexual conquests, a new costume) without having to move substantially out of unconscious living. On the other hand is the intent to stay conscious about being out for the rest of your life in order to utilize the endless challenges to your authenticity as endless opportunities for healing. Only you can know what your true intent is, and you can only know that by listening to what is going on in your own head.

Nobody can make the argument that this is easy, or that they don't embody both intents. I certainly do—it's very easy for me to be out to another gay man I'm hot for, but it's a considerable effort with a straight man I can get nothing from. The difference is that without the desire to get something from someone, my desire to be authentic about my sexuality diminishes, and I can easily find myself passively in the closet with that person.

Knowing this I can always challenge myself to be real no matter what so that I never step back into the closet just because it's easy. The point is to keep these intents in mind so that you are always aware of which one is guiding you. That way you can always make a conscious choice to do the best thing that you could possibly do for yourself, which is to make the effort to be authentic about your sexuality whether you can get something from someone or not. The point isn't to make a political statement or convince homophobes that you're just as good, but rather to help heal the part of you that is still judging yourself to be wrong because you are gay.

Of course, we all feel the pressure to recede into the background even once we've come out—to, in a sense, stay where we're told to stay in our neighborhoods or in our bedrooms.

This pressure to recede is exercised in the form of fears—of violence, of repercussions, of offending, of making people uncomfortable—which are instilled in us in adolescence and which so many of us accept as true. But fear only emanates from the unconscious mind, and like all unconscious thoughts it is on an endless journey to prove itself true. So the problem here is that if you have fear in any form—*and homophobia is itself a fear*—then you will indeed see it everywhere because it is your own that you see.

This is a profoundly complex situation that has been given to us, and there are a myriad of rules held personally by millions of gay men that speak to it. Some believe they shouldn't have to come out to anyone because straight people don't have to; that everyone should know they are gay at all times, even the mailman; or that just because they have sex with men doesn't mean they're gay, so there's nothing to come out of. The list goes on.

The problem with rules is that they are like morals—they do your thinking for you. In other words, they block out the very instrument of freedom that coming out strengthens, which is your connection to the part of you that sees infinite possibilities at all times because you are not bogged down by limits. So coming out just to get laid or live the life of a "fabulous" gay man can keep you in a state of darkness almost as deep as the state you were in while you were closeted because your mind will become chained to that programming. There's no reason to judge those choices, though, because there is nothing wrong with them. But there is great reason to see those choices for where they come from, which is a state of fear, and for what they ultimately produce, which is a lot of suffering.

This doesn't mean you can't be gay and out and authentic and also fabulous and getting laid. Quite the contrary. But it does mean that if you are out only to anesthetize your fears by consuming status and gorging on sexual conquests, you will only make your fear, and thereby your pain, grow.

The only way to navigate the endlessness of coming out with the sense of freedom your heart desires (and which all hearts desire) is to never just react in a way that is comfortable or default to old habits, but rather to set as your intent to face what is going on in your mind every time your authenticity as a gay man is challenged. If you do so, you will find that your actions

17

and reactions in regard to coming out or being out will evolve as you evolve and change in different situations (in other words the rules will fly out the window), but your genuine effort to be whole and true within yourself will not. That is your foundation, and that is where your integrity, your wholeness, your authentic power, your self-awareness, your inner Shining City on the Hill will lie.

In this chapter I will give you guidance to help you find and keep your integrity in every stage of the coming out process. And this is important even if you are out or have been out for a very long time, because you might very well just be out in your comfort zone and avoiding people and places that would expose the part of you that is still in hiding. But remember that this is only guidance—only you can know whether or not you're ready for the truth.

Coming Out to Yourself

I have been attracted to men since I felt my first sexual impulses, but I did not fully accept and acknowledge to myself that I was gay until I was sixteen.

At that time, in 1986, I had been dating a beautiful young girl named Sharon from a neighboring high school. When we met and began seeing each other I was ecstatic because I thought I was in love with her. Though I certainly did come to love her very much, I was not "in love" as I thought. Rather I was ecstatic because I thought my relationship with her meant I must be straight after all. At that age I easily confused this sense of relief and excitement at the idea that I might be straight with being in love. And it was a powerful illusion.

But this illusion began to fall apart very quickly. Six weeks or so into our relationship she went on vacation with her family, and by myself again, my sexual fantasies about men went into full gear. I tried to repress them but to no avail. I broke up with her shortly after under some kind of bogus pretense and descended into a deep depression. It was there that I faced reality and said to myself for the first time, "I'm gay." There was no going around it.

Though this moment was marked by depression and grief, and I would not embrace it and come out to the world for eight more years, it was a very critical step because it was the first time I, even if unwillingly, was forced to face what my awareness and experience had been telling me my whole life: that I was sexually attracted to men and not sexually attracted to women.

I had become aware in middle school that I was sexually attracted to other boys—my locker-room fantasies of my middle school PE coach were enough to clue me in on that, but I did not live in a world that had room for the idea that some boys were attracted to boys and that was normal and fine and perfect just the way it was. And there was active verbiage from the world around me that being gay was abnormal, not fine and totally imperfect, and gays were to be sniffed out and put in their place. How in the world at ten years old could I have fought that? So I believed it, too. But believing it didn't change my sexual nature, and so I began to create a system of denial and separation from it, which was how and when I first stepped into the closet. In my journals, I referred to my sexuality ominously and in all caps as "THE PROBLEM."

At some point I laid all my hopes on a belief I probably picked up on television that my sexual attraction for men was a phase. I also thought that if I could create an outer package that fit the "straight" stereotype I could re-create my insides, so in the meantime I worked hard on that. But my big hope lay in another wrong idea I picked up from somewhere that sex with a woman could fix me. I also tried simply to repress my sexual desires for men and force myself to fantasize about women. And when the word "faggot" entered the picture as the worst, most slanderous, demeaning and dehumanizing word that was uttered by one boy to another, I became even more withdrawn—an Anne Frank in the attic of my own being, only I had to hide from myself, too.

In addition to my hopes were many ignorant and fear-based beliefs that pushed me to reject what was so obviously real about myself. I believed that I couldn't possibly be gay because I would go to hell; I wasn't like the tragic gay figures I saw on television; I was a Christian; I didn't choose it; I was not willing to admit this to anyone; and more to the point, I couldn't be gay because I wanted to have a "normal" life, and gay people were not normal.

With 100 percent of my faith invested in this "reality," in my teenage mind being gay meant my life was destined for tragedy. I asked myself countless times, "Why me?" and asserted to myself endlessly that it just wasn't fair. As I say, I felt shocked by my very own being. Naturally, with this belief system set firmly in my mind, going into the closet was the only way I could survive the shock and live with the terrible news that I was sexually attracted to men—that I was a "faggot," and through no choice of my own.

If this describes your situation, you must be at the place where you are at least willing to consider that you might be sexually attracted to men and not to women. No matter what, you are surely seeking peace and clarity. Of course, that's what we all want in every situation. The way to achieve it, though, is not to deny what is real about you or to try to change it, but rather to set your intent to be true to yourself, to make a real effort to search deep inside, and to willingly accept what you find when you look there.

Take a Journey Inward

If you are sexually attracted to men, and conversely, not sexually attracted to women, then the reality of your sexual orientation should be clear to you. This seems pretty easy to get at—after all, it doesn't take a therapist or a self-help book to alert you when you are turned on by someone. But because the very fact of being attracted to the same sex is contradictory to so many of our belief systems, and because even in this age people are assumed to be straight until proven otherwise, you might have set up an intricate system of denial to block you from acknowledging something even your body alerts you in unmistakable ways is true about you.

The word "gay" is so loaded with connotations and meanings that have nothing to do with your sexual preference that the matter can become still more confused. In this state, "I'm not into the theater, so I can't be gay" can seem, somehow, a rational belief.

The fact is that it is so much easier to deny something that can't be directly and superficially observed than something that can. You can successfully deny that you are gay, but you cannot successfully deny that you are Asian. But denying that you are gay is no less insane. The thing is, you can't "see" someone else's sexual preference (at best it can only be implied) nor can you see your own by looking in the mirror. The only person's sexuality that you can truly know is your own, and you can only know it through feeling your feelings and acknowledging what they tell you. That's because what is most essential in life cannot be "seen" with the eyes; it has to be *felt*.

In addition to beliefs that have clouded your self-knowledge, you may be afraid of what's there, and that's where the struggle will also take place. This can be an extremely stressful situation. I don't suggest that you must eradicate your fear, but rather that you disengage your faith in your fears. After all, your fears do nothing for you but wall you off into a narrow, little prison cell. Once you see this, you can still be quite afraid, but you will no longer really believe in your fear because you are beginning to learn that your fears are never real, and they do not serve your interest. And that is when you will find that you are indeed brave enough to examine what is inside of you, become liberated from the fears that seemed so real, *and find that the truth was not at all what you were afraid it was.*

The first step in this journey is to explore your beliefs. You may have entire walls of beliefs that are so immense and so real that they rise before you in every direction, all the way up to the sky so that they even block out all light. You must first see them *as* beliefs and *as* fears for these walls standing between you and the truth of your perfect self to come crashing down into the pile of nothing that they really are.

Believe me, I know that this wall can seem as high as it is real to you. A guy I went out with a few times from Florida named Shawn stayed in the closet and didn't even allow himself to masturbate until he was thirty years old because he was a member of a strict religious sect, and he believed that being gay was a sin. To him, this was not a belief or a fear, but reality—raw, unchangeable, unquestionable reality. But by the time he hit thirty he had finally suffered enough to question his beliefs, and in doing so he began to see them as beliefs, nothing more . . . and not his religion's beliefs, but his own. (After all, a "religion" cannot have beliefs—only an individual can.) Upon doing so, the walls began to crash, and he became awash in the truth about himself. That is when he came out to himself and to the world and began to actually live and to be the full and complete sexual being that he was made to be.

As long as you hold on to the idea that your fears about what being gay means cannot be questioned because they are real, you will not be able to regain even one ounce of power over yourself or your life. Walk through these fears with faith that you yourself can in no way be diminished by the questioning and releasing of a belief, and you will indeed find yourself ready to take the journey out of prison and into freedom.

Ask Yourself Why You Believe You Can't Be Gay

So ask yourself what it is that you believe. Do you believe that you can't be gay because you want to be straight? Because you didn't choose it? Because if you pretend to be straight it will eventually come to pass? Because you are a real man, and real men are not gay? Because you have not met the right girl yet? Because you don't *want* to be gay? Because there are no gay men in your ethnic group, religion, or from your region of the world? Because you are nothing like gay people you know or see on TV? Because it would mean you were weak? Because you have a girlfriend or a wife or a child? Because accepting it would be against God's will?

I could spoon-feed you a million suggestions, but only you can discover what makes up your personal belief system. The process is very simple, and it begins by saying to yourself, "I believe I can't be gay because . . ." and filling in everything that comes to mind, whenever it comes to mind.

It may take a while—unconscious thoughts are often like the house in your neighborhood you've walked by a million times but somehow never looked at. Becoming aware of what you've never looked at requires that you be on full wakeful alert on your daily walks up and down your street. Instead of daydreaming about what should be there, or what's going on elsewhere, so that you are not aware of what is right before your eyes *right now*, you stop dreaming, and you look at every house. You force yourself to stay awake and pay close attention to this very moment that you are in.

When you do so, that's when you'll spot your first one and think, "Oh my gosh, in all these years I've *never* noticed that house! How in the world did I never see it? Yet it's been there all along!"

If you wake up and stay awake during every moment of the day you will suddenly begin to see lots and lots of things you never noticed. You might be quite stunned at what and who has been living in the neighborhood of your mind, and what they've been doing to your life.

It isn't easy because these parasitical beliefs become entrenched in your system and thereby function as a part of you.

A close friend of mine had an astonishing discovery of what was living in the neighborhood of his mind while I was writing this book. He, too, had grown up in an extremely religious home that condemned homosexuality, but by the time I knew him he was absolutely one of the most out and openly gay people I'd ever met. And he was certain he had left all of that religiously justified self-hatred behind. So was I. But after lots of conversations with me exploring the source of an inexplicable strain of self-destructive behavior, he discovered that he still had a belief functioning in his mind that he was going to literally be crucified for being gay. He thought that coming out of the closet and leaving his religion had rid him of this belief, but underneath all the fabulous gay superstar attire, he still believed he had sinned against God by being gay and was going to pay the price. And in believing this, he was indeed paying a very hefty price because he himself extracted that price with his own beliefs.

Put Those Beliefs on Trial

As with my close friend, just because you can't see a thought doesn't mean it isn't there, it just means you may not be aware of it, which is what "unconscious" means. So once you have come up with your list as to why you can't be gay (and you might want to write them down) next you must question those beliefs.

Whatever your reasons are, keep in mind that they are just beliefs, and you are the one who either gives them life or takes away their life. Without them you can experience a state of unclouded awareness. Keep in mind that this state of unclouded awareness is something that you have already experienced. As a child, before you had beliefs, you were utterly present and accepted everything for how it was in that moment. In that state you would have thought nothing about two men holding hands or living together. It was the belief systems you were indoctrinated into later and that you chose to agree with that created the judgment you have against men who love and have sex with one another. It was later on that you wound up judging yourself. And the way out of this judgment against yourself is through the process of questioning.

The main question to ask yourself is this: do any of the beliefs that I have that I can't possibly be gay have anything to do with the gender that I am attracted to? If you then respond with another belief, such as "I know it is against God because my minister [or mullah, or priest, or rabbi or father or coach] says so," ask yourself again, does what anyone else says cause or change whom you are sexually attracted to? If the answer is no, then you must be willing to let go of that belief; otherwise, you are literally doing the insane, which is to reject what *is*, not to mention squandering your life energy on a lie about yourself that hurts you. Put all of your beliefs on trial in such a way, and you will slowly gain control over your mind and begin to create your life consciously according to your will.

Allow Yourself to Feel What You Feel

Once you have disempowered enough of your belief systems to begin to connect with the true knowledge about yourself, you must now begin to wake up during moments of sexual arousal. This is crucial. Without unfounded beliefs and fears in your way, you can actually perceive *what is* in a state of acceptance and sanity.

The thing about the nature of what is actually real beneath your beliefs and fears is that it doesn't require any thinking and it doesn't need you to believe it—you can believe all day that the world is flat but that doesn't make it flat. And the world doesn't need you to believe that it is round to be round. Similarly, you can believe all day that you are straight but it doesn't make you straight, and you don't need to believe that you are straight or gay in order to be either one—you just are. The point of this exercise is to just see what you are and do the sane thing, which is to accept it.

I know a guy named Michael who has made it clear in every way possible that he is sexually attracted to men—namely, he's always hitting on my friend Scott. Michael has even gone as far as finding an excuse to spend the night with Scott, and then make moves on him in the middle of the night. But after Michael is through he acts as if he has been asleep and doesn't know what happened. Then he begins talking about women and how much he can't wait to get married to one.

This is what is called a split consciousness—part of him is utterly aware that he is hot for Scott, and that is the part that arranges the scenarios in which they wind up in bed together. The other part is so removed from what is happening that he might as well be on another planet. In a way, he is indeed deeply asleep, though not in the way he's telling himself. At this level, it is quite insane, and I feel great compassion for the guy. But I understand that he is in such a state of denial that blocking his perceptions of even the extremely obvious is the only way he can get up the next day and live with himself because his beliefs make it impossible for him, as of yet, to accept who he is.

This may sound familiar to you. But you are not powerless to change it, because once you let go of the beliefs that block your perceptions you will be clear enough to discern what is true, and it will be unambiguous to you. In doing that you will be able to see what actually *is*, and do the sane thing, which is to accept it.

So, as a practice, choose to stay conscious in moments of sexual arousal. Make a choice to observe and note what you find sexually exciting, and also in turn what you do not. Being unclouded by belief, you will slowly bring consciousness and light to your inner sexual reality, and with it clarity and acceptance.

The last step is to move consciously into a state of willful acceptance of the truth—not of what you believe, but with what you have seen and experienced yourself. But the act of seeing what is and accepting it is a process, so give yourself time. It is most likely not urgent that you come to realization this second. A gradual approach to the truth will strengthen the intent to know more and weaken the desire to hide, and eventually you can cross over.

So ask yourself what your intent is right now. Is it to hide from yourself? Bring that to the surface. Then ask yourself if that is indeed what you truly want, given that this road has never brought you more than a fleeting, and profoundly vulnerable, sense of happiness. If hiding from yourself is not truly your heart's desire, then create a new intent to discover yourself and accept what you find. That is all you need to do, and if you do create this intent, you will discover what is inside of you, and in doing so you will find the happiness, clarity and love that you were seeking all along.

Coming Out to Others

It was a long, long time after I came out to myself that I was ready to come out to anyone else. Realizing and accepting that I was gay did not, at first, compel me to relinquish my grip on all my negative beliefs about what it meant to be gay. My need to feel normal, to feel loved, and to have a full and fulfilling life were honest, but I was under the misconception that the only way to fulfill these needs was to look like I thought everyone was supposed to look, and an essential element to that was being heterosexual.

In addition, I felt that there was nothing to come out to. I saw no out gay men nor representations of gay men that I identified with or wanted to be like. And for many of those years I had a story line running in my mind that if I did come out I would no longer be loved and accepted by the world that I knew. As a result, I was in a position where the only way for me to achieve my goals was to pretend I wasn't gay even though I knew I was.

Slowly, through the end of my teens and into my early twenties, the belief that this route would bring me fulfillment began to erode. I eventually did achieve the kind of "popularity" and normality I craved within a context of supposed heterosexuality on the outside, but I was still broken and disintegrated on the inside. I was extremely sexually frustrated, and I was sick of lying—especially to close friends, like my friend Liza who would try to bring it up out of love and concern, and I would go running in the other direction. That was such a wake-up call, but I insisted on pressing the snooze button by running away from it every time because I was so scared.

I know that a lot of gay men go through a transition period of pressing the snooze button before they decide to wake up and come out. There was a guy I knew at a magazine named Russ whom everyone assumed was gay and out. In response he would make loud proclamations about the fact that he was not gay, and they got louder over time. Once people stopped speaking to him as if he were an out gay man, he went silent on the issue for months. Then one day, lo and behold, he showed up at a work party with a guy. So basically people had been inadvertently trying to pull him out before he was ready, but he admitted afterward that it was an alarm going off that he needed to heal his situation. And the only person not relieved was his gay boss who had a big crush on him and was devastated that he'd already found someone else.

It was also my increasingly extreme discomfort with my inauthentic life that pushed me incrementally in the direction of making the decision to come out. First I decided that I needed to. Then I decided to at least take the step of no longer actively lying about my sexuality. From that step slowly grew the intent to actually come out. I didn't know how I was going to do it. But never mind that, or the fact that I still didn't think I had anything to go to once I came out—my discomfort with my daily existence was enough to make me think just being honest was enough motivation to make the leap.

So with my intent set to come out I simply waited, on some level knowing that a route would have to present itself. And it did with the chance to publish the essay in *Details* magazine.

After the piece was accepted and had gone to press, I went into a state of denial over what was about to happen in my life. I had set wheels in motion that I could not stop. I remember one time on the subway, as the day of reckoning drew close, I almost fainted as I moved into the twilight zone of awareness of the fact that I was gay, only knowing that this time I would not be able to get out of it.

Then one day in September of 1994, I came home to my small basement apartment in Boston and found copies of the magazine that had been mailed to me. I was sitting in my room with a copy opened up on my lap very still and in a state of shock when my straight friend Tom who had moved up to Boston with me (and who had read the magazine before I did) came in the room quietly. I looked up at him. He sat down on the bed and hugged me. I cried. And that was that. I was out.

The reactions from friends and family were the polar opposite of all of my fears. Over the next few weeks I literally had to erect a chart on my wall in my kitchen to keep track of everyone

I knew who'd called to congratulate me.

For me, it was the perfect remedy. I was able to write what amounted to a letter full of honesty, love and truth to my loved ones about my life, and to get it done in one swoop. In addition, I had editors editing out any negativity in my story in the form of blame or anger so that I only showed my very best side. And once the deed was done, there was no turning back, so no amount of fear could get me to reverse position and stay huddled in a state of paralysis.

Of course this one-fell-swoop, public-outing method isn't right for everyone. For a lot of men, incremental outing is the best way because coming out to their sister feels safe and good, but it may take years before they are ready to face their fears over their father's reaction. Or vice versa. For others, just showing up at home with a guy on their arm is the right way because it allows people to figure it out on their own and bring it up when they are ready. The point is that there is no one-size-fits-all method, but the right method for you will present itself as soon as you are ready.

What was astounding for me was that, after the article came out, what I had built up in my mind as a nightmare scenario turned out to be a beautiful celebration. I felt relief and wholeness on a scale I simply couldn't have imagined. The fact that my catharsis, revelation and bravery resonated with the people in my life, regardless, and that I received warm congratulations was a wonderful perk and taught me many lessons about the power of truth to transform situations and its deep appeal to the human spirit. But it was just gravy, because the meal was in feeling my own acceptance, which is the only acceptance I can ever feel anyway.

This was, of course, my experience. But the essential elements to it are the same with most gay men—the discontentment with life in the closet, the incremental steps in the direction of truth, setting the intent to come out, and seeing the opportunity and following through—and will continue to be that way until society as a whole no longer functions under an assumption of heterosexuality.

Take the First Step to Coming Out to Others by Removing Beliefs That Disempower You

Just as you had roadblocks in your own mind to coming out to yourself, you might have placed barriers between you and the idea of living authentically as an out gay person. If this is so, the process is the same: you release yourself from defending those barriers at all costs and then disassemble your belief system, which gives you the false impression that you do not have the power to live an authentic life as an out gay man that is fulfilling and perfectly right for you.

Stop believing in the movie in your mind that says you can't live a perfect life as a gay man, and you will connect to the awesome power you have to live any way you like.

So begin by questioning your "reality," by bringing to the surface any beliefs you have that you cannot come out to other people. Maybe you believe that if you do come out you will have to live a certain kind of life you see on TV; that your parents will reject you; that you will never feel accepted again; that your loved ones can't handle the truth; that people will see you as a "faggot," and you can't live like that; or that you will somehow have to give up everything you cherish. Whatever your beliefs are, bring them to the surface and take a close look.

Let Go of What You Are Afraid Will Happen When You Come Out and Be Open to What Does

Whatever your beliefs are about what would happen if you came out, you must realize this: you do not know what will happen. It is your fears that are so real to you, not a future reality that you have the power to detect. That's what I mean by the movie playing in your mind—even if it's a terrible movie you still believe in it because you created it. But that doesn't mean it's real.

What's real is that you have no idea what people feel or think about you now or what they will feel and think later—it is only your own thoughts and feelings that you think and feel. It may seem as if someone else thinks you're a faggot, but it can only be you who feels like a faggot. If you do not feel like a faggot, the term "faggot" does not exist for you. End of story.

Realize this and you will realize the end of the reign of power your own internal, personal abuse system has over you that is trying to keep you down. Looking at the unconscious self in this way, it is just like an external abuse situation—as the abused you take it because you believe it's true and you deserve it. Realize it isn't true and that you don't deserve it and the power the abuser has over you goes away.

Realize That Your Power Lies in Changing Yourself, Not in Controlling Others

All of this boils down to realizing where your power lies, and where it doesn't. Your power does not lie in controlling others— you really don't know how anyone else is going to feel about you coming out of the closet, and trying to control that will give you a sense of powerlessness.

But you do have the power to love yourself entirely for exactly how you are, and to realize the absolute perfection of your entire being, most especially inclusive of your sexual nature. That is true power. That is strength. Focusing on other people's perceived lack of acceptance is a giant distraction from the fact that it is only ever your own acceptance or rejection that you feel. Believing it is other people who cause you to feel rejected is your way of avoiding responsibility and of keeping yourself locked in a prison of endless suffering, because you will never be able to change anyone else. You must refocus your attention on what is going on inside of you in order to connect to your true power.

Have Faith That You've Got the Power to Create Any Kind of Life You Want as an Out Gay Man

You must also have trust in yourself and the cosmos that you will be able to reorder your life to suit the authentic you. You have probably already done this in one way or another—picked one place to live, one friend to have, one class to take over others because they suited you. This power you have to do as you please does not come to a stop when it comes to creating your life as an out gay man. You've got the power to do whatever you like. It will take exploring and investigating and experimenting. It will also take time. But everything does. And thank God, because after all, that is how we go about learning about ourselves.

The point is that behind all of your own fears and limits and ideas is your power. All you have to do is walk through them to access it. And you'll find you have more power than you ever could have imagined.

Prepare Yourself to Make a New Statement

The most important element of actually coming out of the closet is the statement it makes about where you are with your sexuality. While in the closet, the statement you made was either an outright lie ("I'm straight; I'm not gay.") or simply, "No comment." Once you are sick enough of the deception, the need to shed this false layer by just getting it all out in the open can become overwhelming. Nevertheless, though you are delivering the information to other people actively for the first time, it is still primarily about you, not them. In essence, the healthy statement you're making when you come out of the closet is that you're now okay enough with your sexuality to talk about it and to begin living a life in accordance with it.

The first thing to do once you are ready to start making your way down the road toward freedom and honesty is to clean yourself up of negativity. So try this: rehearse your new statement of honesty about your sexuality. You can do this verbally by yourself, write it down, say it to a video camera or just say it to yourself in your mind . . . whatever works for you. Acknowledge that you are simply practicing and take the pressure off. I'm not suggesting that you put on a lavender sweater, look in the mirror and be all Stuart Smalley about it—though, honestly, you could do worse. What I am suggesting is that you rehearse it first alone and let it all just come out exactly as it is in you right now.

Take a Close Look at What Comes Out

Afterward, deconstruct what comes out, and make a point of looking for negative emotions, such as blame, guilt, judgment, fear, anger, vindictiveness and aggression. The primary reason you must work to clean yourself up of these negative emotions is that they emanate from your unconscious self. If they are there you will project them onto others and then either blame them for these emotions or try to change them so you don't feel these emotions. And you will not be able to see what is actually there to be seen in their reactions.

Also, if you come from a state of fear, that is what you will engender in others. Your whole point in coming out is to leave fear behind, so why in the world would you couch your freedom from fear in fear? Though being afraid will make sense to your internal abuser trying to keep you in the prison of fear and pain, it does not make sense to a conscious mind always working for liberation into sanity, opportunity and love.

After you have worked on cleaning yourself up of your own fear and negativity, try your rehearsal again. This time focus on simply being honest, with a super-focus on yourself.

Let Go of Your Expectations, Good and Bad, of How People Will Respond

In fact, you should have no expectation of response because that is a setup for disaster if people do not meet your expectations. No matter how close they are, their reactions still have nothing to do with you but rather everything to do with where they are in their own journeys toward self-love and awareness. Letting go of attaching to or predicting the reactions of others like you'd let go of something extremely hot that would burn you is a good approach because they are both just as dangerous.

Rather, simply focus on delivering your message with love from your own heart, for that will help melt away distance and fear, and connect your listener to the universal point of your story, which every person on the Earth can relate to, which is your personal journey toward happiness and fulfillment.

If they support you, that's great, and you can celebrate. If they don't, it is just a reflection of their own desire to keep themselves down. And that is the fact of the matter for everyone who does not support your coming out: at its essence it has nothing to do even with homophobia—that's just the surface programming. Rather, it has everything to do with their own limits, which, through your actions, you are proving do not actually exist. Maybe they'll be inspired; maybe they'll be threatened. Either way, it has nothing to do with you. Realize that and you truly have nothing to be afraid of.

Don't Weigh Yourself Down with the Future

Finally, prepare to be open to what happens next. You do not have to load yourself down with what is going to happen in your life for the next fifty years as a result of coming out, or answer every question people may have about gay men. All you need to do is prepare to do your best, be as honest as you can, and have a heart full of love for yourself, and you will be fine.

Take the Big Step: Intent

The first and most essential part of coming out is to simply set an intent to do so. Though the buildup to a new intent can be a big struggle, actually setting one is a wonderful expression of your personal power and a great opportunity to take the stress off yourself and allow the universe to give you the opportunities you need to fulfill your desire.

I know making references to Jesus can be loaded for a lot of people, especially gay people because so much negative energy toward us has been done in his name, but that is not his fault; he is long gone and can't defend himself. However, if you look beyond that into what Jesus said, he really had it down about how the universe works and the nature of the self and just how powerful you truly are, especially when it comes to the power of your intention.

In his Sermon on the Mount, which he made just to the people who got him, Jesus gave very clear instruction on this matter when he said, "Ask, and it shall be given to you; seek, and ye shall find; knock, and it shall be opened unto you." He meant that God, the All, the Cosmos, whatever you want to call the single all-powerful force behind creation that is the essence of your being, will make opportunities and ideas available to you once you've decided you are ready for them. The strength of your intention is the determining factor of the outcome.

This is also the fundamental meaning behind the philosopher Joseph Campbell's conclusion that the "hero gets the adventure he's ready for." Once you're ready for something, it will come to you. And his observation is absolutely applicable to you in this situation: you are a hero for coming out, and you are now ready for a new journey.

Don't Worry About How You're Going to Do It

You do not need to fret over how and when you are going to come out for the first time to someone else. Also, chances are it is not urgent that you come out immediately, so be patient with yourself.

What this also means is that any preconceived ideas about

how to do it—in the form of a full-on Broadway production, a group e-mail, twenty different private discussions or subtle hints—might bear no relation to what opportunities actually appear before you. You can start with those closest to you or start with strangers. You can write letters and e-mails or simply start responding honestly to questions and assumptions. You can even start living your new life now, and let others figure it out—after all, this is exactly your right as a human being, so if you just want to go ahead and start dating openly or referring to other men as cute or hot, then do that. Just be open to the channels that will be offered to you in any given moment. Remember, I could never have predicted the way it worked for me, and it was so much more genius than anything I could have come up with on my own.

You have many freedoms at hand. You can even avoid labels if you like. As long as you are honest about being sexually attracted to men, you're good to go—just be careful that you aren't blowing up more smoke, which is the real story behind men who sleep with men but who deny they are gay.

You don't have to "spare" people either—in fact doing so indicates that you have a pretty low opinion of them, and after all, it's your fear that you sense, not theirs. And you don't do anyone any favors by not being authentic in their presence. In fact that's the worst thing you can do because you give them no opportunity to take inspiration from your growth and grow themselves.

Finally, have faith. You may not be able to imagine how you're going to feel afterward, but know that you will feel a huge burden lift and will begin to discover the bliss of authenticity for yourself.

Coming Out in Difficult Circumstances

Though coming out is most definitely first and foremost about you, often there are circumstances in which gay men have become very invested in their "straight" lives. In these cases the elements to coming out can require a great deal of extra consideration.

For instance, you might have involved other people in your closeted life in the form of a girlfriend or wife. In this case you are going to have a lot of work to do in the area of acknowledging fully why you entered into the relationship, apologizing and expressing your love. Amends are most definitely in order, as well.

However, as much as the truth may hurt you and your female partner, it can't possibly be as destructive as a relationship founded in large part on a very big lie, which is also keeping both of you from having a truly fulfilling relationship. And of all the billions of reasons behind the billions of heterosexual breakups in this world, one partner being gay is as good a reason as it gets.

Of course, it gets a lot more involved if you are married with children. In this case you have to weigh further the needs of your children versus the initial destabilization in the family structure that will take place by acknowledging your sexuality. Any way you slice it, your responsibilities to your family will not change as a result of coming out of the closet—you may no longer be someone's husband or boyfriend if you come out, but you will not stop being someone's father, nor do you have to stop loving and doing right by your former partner.

In that sense, the well-being of your family should be as big a concern as your own—and trust that your authenticity can only serve the interests of your children who need you as an example when it comes to their own journeys toward authenticity, whether they are gay or straight. And remember the power of intention: set your intent on being open to the route most likely to result in a healthy reorganization and let the universe unfold the possibilities for you.

I know a gay guy named Eduardo who was married and had a son with his wife. Since coming out and getting divorced, he has remained an incredibly devoted father and continues to bend over backward to do everything to support his ex-wife. It is true that she is still not accepting of the fact that he is gay, but what I admire most about Ed is that he does not take it personally nor burden himself with guilt over his decision to come out. The fact is that he was gay all along, and his acceptance of it was the best thing that he could do for his relationship with his wife, which was, after all, based on a lie and is now based on truth. He can't control her lack of desire to accept what is true, but he does his part, and that's all that he can do. The fact that he can see this is what has made it possible for him to remain an integral part of his own family and be out of the closet at the same time. Just remember that there are infinite possibilities; you just have to let go of the fearful and limiting outcomes in your mind in order to begin to see them.

You might also still be living at home and vulnerable to potential violence from a family member or at school. If you believe that you might be in physical danger from a family member or kids at school, or that you might even be kicked out of your home, it may be that coming out publicly at this time is not the best idea. If this is the case, it doesn't mean that you stay in denial, or that you can't reach out elsewhere to friends, and/or to gay organizations. It might be that the wisest thing is to set your intent on getting out from under the control of dangerous people before you begin to live openly as a gay person. Stay conscious and you'll know what to do.

If you are employed in genuinely homophobic environs or involved in a conservative religious organization, some serious life reorganization is also probably called for. If this is the case, being gay and out is going to shake things up. But they need shaking up. And trust that you certainly won't be the first gay man in your field to come out—there are more marines, priests, conservative politicians, high school principals and football players who've come out of the closet and found lives that are fulfilling to them than you could ever shake a stick at. So trust me, you're in good company.

Though there is no way anyone can "protect" you from the choices that you are going to have to make, know that protection is pointless, because these choices *are* your journey toward self-realization. So if you set your intent on creating honesty and integrity in your life, living consciously and being open to the inspiration that will come to you, you will find the freedom you long for.

Take the Continuous Opportunities for Coming Out as Continuous Opportunities to Heal

Coming out of the closet for the first time is a lot like turning thirty. Your first thought is that you made it, whew, now it's over. But then you turn thirty-one.

As every out gay man knows, it is the same once you've come out of the closet. After you've made your first big leap you are so proud and so relieved. Then one day soon you find yourself in a new environ—a new job, a new city, a new apartment building—only to discover that you are living under the assumption of straightness again. And it still doesn't end there, because even the service guy at the gas station is making comments to you about women, expecting a heterosexual response. Suddenly it's like you've been shoved back in the closet without realizing it.

This is a fact of life for the out gay man. Unfortunately, very often our reactions to the challenge of the ongoing coming out process lack the conscious effort and authenticity that were summoned up for the initial coming out. And this makes sense.

For a lot of gay men, the attitude is that once you're out to all the important people and you're living a life in accordance with your sexuality, who cares if they know at work or at the grocery store? For others, the opposite reaction is called up. Either fueled by a sense of political activism or by a belief that being gay is the dominant part of their being, they feel that everyone they encounter should know they are gay, and they should know it now regardless of who, what, where, when or how.

It's no wonder gay men wouldn't want to cope with constantly having to come out, and why so many sequester themselves in gay ghettos where they are always assumed gay and are never challenged again. After all, and I know this from personal experience, it makes life so easy.

But to not continue to put the same effort into the ongoing challenge to your authenticity as an out gay man is to miss out on the opportunities for healing that continuously coming out offers. Instead, you open yourself up to unconscious living. This is because, any way you slice it, you're not making conscious decisions in individual circumstances but, rather, choosing to let your unconscious fears and beliefs create your life for you. And by creating your life unconsciously your goal is no longer about your integrity—it's about making your lifestyle easy or mistaking political statements for personal growth.

The fact is that life is a constant process of coming out of what you aren't and into what you really are. As a gay man, your sexual preference is one integral element of this process, and as you go on and evolve in this life, the challenge of being out with integrity is always being bumped up to the next level. Ignoring this challenge is no less significant to the process of shedding false layers of your identity than the first time you came out to yourself.

Stay Flexible—Don't Get Rigid

As I've said before, there are no absolute rules of external behavior in terms of your level of "outness" in the world. The challenge is to wake up and watch yourself, so you can always create conscious intents to live in truth. And to do this you must learn to distinguish between the voices in your own head and other people's voices.

For instance, one time I was in a very small locker room with about six men with whom I train in the Brazilian martial art capoeira, all of whom were in various states of undress. One of them spoke up and mentioned that he had seen me on television talking about an article I'd written. It was on a gay topic, and I paused before I answered. The room went quiet waiting for a response, and I was so sure that they would be uncomfortable with my answer, given where we were and that we were all half naked. But then I realized that it was my own discomfort I felt. After all, whose feelings do I feel but my own? So I walked through that fear and answered honestly, and it turned out that *I* was definitely the one with the problem, not them.

Realizing this helped me heal my fear. Not taking the opportunities situations like these offer is like carrying a closet with you everywhere you go. If a stranger asks you if you have a girlfriend, and you still have fears and self-rejections you haven't dealt with that result in an unconscious intent to hide, this question, even if you've been out for twenty years, can suddenly make you go running for the closet.

But if you deal with those self-rejections you can rid yourself of them. In a state of self-love and acceptance and recognition of your perfection, you can then say, "No, I don't, but in my case it would be a boyfriend," as easy as you would tell someone that you were from California not Ohio. That's exactly how I play it anytime anyone assumes I'm straight *because* I call my fears what they are, and then I face them. Not in a state of fear, fear doesn't exist for me. You have all the power to do the same.

There is no denying that the ongoing coming out process requires a great deal of effort. That's because you didn't kill in one swoop every single unconscious fear about yourself when you came out. Many still linger—believe me, they do. But once you're officially out you begin to mask them with justifications for staying in the closet situationally, such as that you would lose money if you came out at work; that certain straight people in your life simply wouldn't be able to handle it; that it's sexier to seem straight; that you aren't "gay," you just like to do it with men; or that it's too much effort to come out all the time.

You might notice that these beliefs sound very much like the beliefs of a closeted person. That's because they are, and just as with a totally closeted person, they represent an acute case of self-rejection. And this is the very uncomfortable truth behind the trend among many gay men to live gay sexual lives but to not identify as such: underneath it all is a searing lack of self-love. And there is nothing hot about that when it is seen for what it is.

In order to turn all these challenges into opportunities for self-realization, you must create an intent to be authentic and conscious in every setting you find yourself in which there is an active or passive assumption of your straightness. And the benefits of allowing this light to come in are enormous. The more clear and conscious you are, the less fearful you will be, the more you will give yourself the love and acceptance that you deeply desire, and the more able over time you will be to simply observe the illusions of the world, even as they pertain to you, and help out those around you who are in their grip.

This is because the continued process of coming out fully in the service of yourself can also eventually be done in the true service of others, and this will help you transmute an anxious, fearful and confused inner condition into one of peace, clarity and freedom, which you will then be able to offer to everyone you come into contact with. That way you'll not just be ready for the truth, you'll be its messenger, too.

3

You Are No More "Gay" Than You Were "Straight"

Nothing real can be threatened.
Nothing unreal exists.

—*A Course in Miracles*

There was a point when I was about a year into immersing myself in New York's gay life that, utterly enamored and riveted by it, and finding it so deliciously all-consuming, I heard an inner voice say, "I want nothing to do anymore with anything that isn't gay."

Even in the rush of my new gay life, this totally gay vision for myself came as a little bit of a shock to me. After all, I had spent my entire life up until that point thinking of gay men as shadowy and tragic, and I had done everything in the world to put a distance between myself and that image.

But now, having seen the modern gay world with my own eyes, I was feeling the exact opposite: not only did gay men not seem "shadowy" at all to me (but rather just human beings like anyone else), so many of the gay men I saw on the streets of New York seemed impossibly beautiful, confident, sexy and sophisticated. In fact, in some ways, they actually seemed *superior* to straight people. And imagine my shock when I saw doormen at clubs lining straight people up down the block like they were cattle while gay men were escorted in like celebrities! This seemed like a truly bizarre turn of events.

Taking a look at this gay micro-universe, which was ready to satisfy every part of me that had starved for so long, I was sold. I decided that I most definitely wanted from the gay world what my friend Darren sums up as "membership" in the club. I wanted in.

So once I finally let go of my preppy, "straight" frat boy costume, which could no longer get me what I wanted, I found myself chomping at the bit to don a "gay" one. As with my frat boy facade, it was quite logical to me that engineering the right gay costume was the means by which I could get my membership and everything in the gay world—sex, attention, approval, fulfillment—that I could see truly awesome potential for.

Of course, underlying this quest was my endless search for perfection, which I was now absolutely sure was only dished out to hot, beautiful gay men.

Engineering My Character, and the Search for Gay Heaven

I recall the exact moment I realized how I was going to get my membership. I was at a famous gay bar in New York with a friend who had been taking me out and showing me the ropes. At that time, in 1995 when I first moved to New York, I was going out a lot (even if going out meant just walking the streets of Chelsea and the Village), but I still felt like I was sitting on the periphery of gay culture. I spent most of my time just looking at gay men with their muscles, their fashion, their fabulousness and their confidence and strategizing how I could get in on what they had. The question was, how do I get my membership? How do I become one of them?

With this question front and center in my brain, I went up to one of the bars to get a drink. And in one moment I got my flash of true gay perfection and the inspiration I was looking for in the form of the bartender.

The one I walked up to was in his late twenties. He was superhandsome with black, wavy hair and a long, muscular torso of the sort I'd only ever seen in porn before. The lighting from beneath the bar gave him a mystical neon glow, which enhanced the sense that it wasn't just about the drinks, the music, the dance floor, or the gay men in the bar—it was about him.

While I waited for him to pour my drink, I gazed on him and fantasized about his perfect life: his sex life must be amazing, every guy must want him, and I'll bet just living in that body must infuse every activity with a powerful sense of fulfillment. And when I looked around the bar and saw crowds of men waiting around in what I could only call subservience to the bartenders, it certainly looked like everyone else agreed. These guys weren't just members of the club, they were princes.

It was in that very moment that I cast a powerful spell on myself that this bartender, and all other gay men like him, had it all. So if I wanted to have it all, I needed to be like them. I needed to be a prince.

So I set out to make this happen. I tripled my efforts at the gym and became hugely muscular (it turns out I had been a gym queen for ten years already, and I didn't even know it!), got a Fifth Avenue haircut, and I threw out all the Polo shirts and Cole Haan loafers and replaced them with vinyl Katharine Hamnett pants and boutique tank tops from Patricia Field. I began to hit every party in New York, Fire Island and Miami Beach and learned how the subculture worked—how to get on the guest list, who the big DJs were, whom to buy drugs from, and how to pick up beautiful men. I then recalibrated my demeanor to mimic the aloofness I saw in bartenders every-where, and I had the finishing touch. During these first few months I was in a real rush because I could not stop thinking about all the amazing sex and parties that were going on that I was missing out on.

When I decided the package was complete enough I pre-sented myself to the owner of that very bar wearing my new costume and asked for a job. He focused the light of his atten-tion on me and proceeded to give me the glowing full-body assessment of approval that I would, as the years went by, become deeply addicted to. I'll never forget it, because when he looked at me that way, I felt truly *powerful*. Talk about morphine—this was a real fix.

Et voilà, in less than a year after my introduction to gay society, my character as a gay bartender was debuted.

How My Gay Character Helped Anesthetize My Pain

Looking back at the time of transition, the most serious shift in my experience was from feeling invisible, excluded and not good enough when I first stepped onto the scene, and, once I'd engineered my new gay image, to gay men shooting piercing rays of acceptance from their eyes. Standing behind the bar, especially, I felt a rush of power over others to give me those laser looks of love, and as a bartender, it was at my discretion to accept them, or not.

And because it seemed to be the perfect antidote to all my fears that I was the despicable outcast character I played in high school, I began to identify completely with this accepted and perfect gay bartender character I was now playing.

Given what was going on in me deep inside, this all makes perfect sense. As an adolescent, the mirror could be a real shock because I did not like, or accept, what I saw. Fourteen years later when I was working at the bar, I would often catch my image in the mirror across the dance floor standing behind the bar with my shirt off and that same neon bar light giving me and my shoulder blades that mystical glow, and I would still be shocked; only this time I would think, "People think *I'm* beautiful!"

This new character was not just played out at the bar. Falling in love with this wonderful idea of me, practically my entire focus shifted over to creating the character of a young, muscular, gay party boy. When I discovered that I wasn't just a boy but a "white boy," I began to play that role, too.

And I played him 'round the clock: I went to fabulous circuit parties; slept with guys who were awesomely gorgeous to me; lived with a famous DJ right off 8th Avenue in the heart of Chelsea (which was great because I always had the best mixed tapes); had homoerotic nudes of myself published in a book; wrote a nightlife column for *HX* magazine; and worked out at a gay gym down the street just swarming with hot, available guys so that a simple workout could often turn into a true romantic adventure.

Strolling down West 21st Street listening to Deborah Cox on my Walkman on the way to some party, I felt just like John Travolta on the way to the club in *Saturday Night Fever,* right down to getting upset when someone would mess up my hair. I felt like I had totally made it into gay heaven. This was it—this really was the answer I had been looking for my whole life.

The Wake-Up Call That Something Was Wrong

There is no doubt that it very often seemed like a fantastic dream come true. Having withheld myself from so much of what I needed to experience in my life, taking a gigantic bite of the lotus of gay life was as sensual as it was thrilling. So many aspects of my personality that I had rejected were released and finally allowed to roam free. I was getting to have crushes, go on dates and sleep with men, walk the streets with no shame about being gay, feel like I was truly at the top of the heap instead of the bottom, and act as "gay" as I wanted—especially now that "gay" to me meant hot and beautiful. To sum it up, I was having the time of my life.

These things seemed like a miracle. And they were exactly what I needed because I was proving that I was more than my fears about myself. The fundamental problem, though, was that just like with my frat boy costume, playing the role of a gay prince did not rid me of my rejected outcast character. In fact, my internal abuser was still whispering in my ear that I was not good-looking enough, that no one wanted to have sex with me, and that I would always be excluded in the end.

And every time this ancient "reality" of mine asserted itself again, I would feel truly schizo.

According to what I "knew," having now become everything that being gay was supposed to mean, I should have had, felt and been everything I had fantasized about in that bartender. Yes, I got a huge rush when my gay character's ideas of myself were reinforced, especially in my truest moments of "gay heaven" at a circuit party in Miami Beach surrounded by beautiful men.

But when that "reality" was threatened—when the guy I met at the party never called me again, when I wasn't given the high-profile shifts at the bar, when I did not wake up in the morning feeling fulfilled just because I had great legs—I could suddenly hear my abuser loud and clear telling me that I was still sitting alone at the unpopular table in the cafeteria, so to speak, and all I had been doing was fantasizing that I'd made it when, in fact, I looked like an ass.

This was a devastating thought to me, if not my worst nightmare of life come true. That's when I would go from John Travolta to Regan in *The Exorcist,* writhing on her bed and babbling obscenities as different demons take over her mind. That's because what I'd really done was transfer my self-rejections from straight prep school boys in the South onto gay party boys in

New York. Not realizing that they were my own rejections of myself, not anyone else's, I was always trying to correct my life externally rather than internally. And thus I would always fail.

After four years of vomiting up green puke on myself and everyone else every time some guy I met in the bathroom of Palladium at seven in the morning didn't call, I could not help but see the endless cycles of depression and misery as a symptom that something was not working. After all, if I was living the gay dream and the dream was not making me happy, there was clearly something wrong with the dream—or to be more specific, my dream. Plus I was going to be thirty soon and the fear of receiving diminishing returns in the looks department from gay men seemed to me like a wall of steel my whole image of myself would crack like an egg on if I didn't make some serious changes.

But it wasn't just the extreme insecurity that was the wake-up call—it was also my behavior and my thoughts. When I took a real look at my "personality," I saw that, in many ways, my mind was not my own.

I observed myself acting like a "queen" if it was expected, or "butch" if I didn't want people to think I was a queen. I blew people off because it was appropriate for a "Cheslea boy" like me to do so. I referred to gay men as "faggots" in order to dress them down. I thought I'd eventually be infected with HIV no matter what I did simply because I was gay. I believed that finding the right man was all about finding the physically perfect person to complement my physicality—and, lord knows, that was not working out. And I turned every gay man into a confirmation machine because the most important aspect of my relationship with any gay man was that he indicate that I was beautiful and perfect.

In short, the reason my mind was not my own was because my gay character was doing all the thinking for me. Like me, I think a lot of gay men are surprised that after they've let go of their straight costume and taken on a gay one they eventually find themselves almost as confined and conflicted as they were before. But because they are indeed gay they do not feel free to question the thoughts that create the limits, no matter how painful the confinement. Convincing people to not question their beliefs is how cults of all kinds keep members enslaved, and I was definitely thinking what the cult was telling me to.

I had lost all interest in anything that wasn't gay because my character could only survive in gay surroundings, and I sometimes found myself thinking of straight people as I used to think of gay people—as "other."

With this thought to cut myself off from any aspect of the world that didn't reflect and reinforce my new "gay" image, I had moved from one pole to its opposite, having at one time rejected everything that was gay, and now rejecting everything that was straight. The commonality between them was an unconscious and sincere belief that each character was the real me, the former based on the idea that "straight" was perfect, the latter on the idea that "gay" was perfect.

Over the next few years, just as I had become unable to live with my phony "straight" identity, I became less and less able to tolerate my phony "gay" one because, the fact was, it wasn't making me happy.

So at the age of twenty-nine, with a great deal of ambivalence I stepped out of character. Stripped of so many of my external reinforcements—I got out from behind the bar, I was no longer at the club every Saturday looking for a guy to tell me I was beautiful, and sans my nightlife column so that I was no longer nightclub royalty—I was forced to turn my attention inward, and that's when I began to see what was really going on with me.

Stepping Out of Character and Finding Heaven Within

Stepping away from gay life and everything external that used to capture my attention, I could suddenly pay attention to what was actually being said in my own head. What I discovered was, in fact, insane, because practically every thought began with either "He thinks I'm gorgeous," or "He thinks I'm pathetic." This is when it occurred to me: how the hell would I know what someone else thinks? I began to realize something profound—that this was *me* thinking I was gorgeous or pathetic. Or more specifically, it was my various characters asserting their reality by projecting their thoughts onto other people.

This is when I began to see that there was no "gay dream" beyond my own. There was no communal experience called the "gay world" to be a member of or to be excluded from. "Gay heaven" didn't exist. And the bodies and the glamour and all of that was not what being gay meant—it was what being gay meant *to me*. My entire conception of gay life and myself as a gay man was only real to me because I believed in it.

By transferring my personal dream onto an imaginary "gay world," it seemed as if it were an external reality that I was seeking out and reacting to. In reality it was a holographic image of a gay world that existed in my head. Gullible to this illusion of my own making, I sought out external power over others to make others feel good about me, when the only person who could make me feel good or bad about myself was me. Allowing the truth of this revelation to sink in, I was able to slowly, day by day, drop the illusion of all my characters and begin to connect with my true self who had brought the characters to life.

This was when I began to see my true power. The fact was

that I had created all of my various characters. And to think I had thought of myself for so much of my life as a powerless victim when in fact I was so powerful that I could, in ten short years, exist as a closeted suburban high school outsider, a popular pseudo-straight collegiate frat boy, and a gay New York City bartender prince! The fundamental flaw was that though I had created them, they were not me and I didn't realize how I was using my power.

I know a guy named Norm who insists that he doesn't fit in gay life because he's "not buff." Never mind that he's a brilliant and great-looking guy who people adore—everywhere he goes there's an aura of exclusion about him, and he feels victimized by it.

But the truth is that this is his power in use—he creates the "outsider" character, and his surroundings comply. Similarly, I had created my own characters, yet I was in fact none of them, and none of them was real. That's why each one was so vulnerable to threat; because only "reality" can be threatened because "reality" is nothing but ideas. What is real cannot be threatened in any way because it does not require an idea of it to exist. I am real because I exist without ideas. My characters were "real" because they need me to believe in them.

But each character did have purpose in my life. I had unconsciously created each of them in order to learn that I was always the accepter and rejecter of myself based on my own conditions, which I was responsible for. Seeing this truth I was able to begin the process of letting them go. I didn't need them any more when I began to make the choice to accept and love myself no matter what. In that state I no longer need to believe that you think I have it all. I know I have it all.

57

Connecting with Who I Am
Behind the Characters

By realizing this, I finally began to find the true way out that I had been searching for all along. In doing so I was no longer giving in to what my character wanted, what it said it needed, what made it happy, and more important, what made it real to me. Looking at it this way, I started to be aware of when it was ruling my behavior.

At first my life began to change in little ways. For instance, I stopped taking it personally if some guy lost interest in me, because I realized I was only upset if it threatened my gay character's perfect idea of me or revealed an inner belief that underneath it all I really was the rejected version of me. No longer boondoggling my life force away by trying to figure out the impossible—what someone else thinks about me—my time, my attention and my energy began to free up.

The changes over the years have been dramatic. I am no longer chained by the fear that if I show you who I truly am underneath my fabulous gay character you're going to see a rejected, undesirable and pathetic person. In a state of self-acceptance I can naturally then extend acceptance to others and focus on giving that.

I can relax with people now, especially gay men. I'm not defensive like I used to be because I have so much less to defend. I can be the real me at any time to the best of my ability, which is as fearless as it is indestructible and has absolutely no limits on love. And this is absolutely true of everyone I come into contact with, and this is absolutely true of you, too.

I even practice it with the role I've created for myself with this book. If I choose to believe that I *am* an enlightened self-help author, a lot can threaten that in the form of my unconscious negativity, which I am still dealing with. And believe me, I deal with a lot just like you because I am just like you. Not believing that I *am* my latest character leaves me free to work hard to expose myself to everyone because I know that "self-help author" is just a role. With nothing to lose I can have a sense of humor about the whole thing—the shift in my life in such a short period of time from preppy, closeted, Southern frat boy to self-centered New York gay party boy to enlightened self-help author is quite funny, you know. It's very Madonna.

In short, the less I identify with my characters, the broader my world becomes.

The True Nature of the Roles We Play

The lesson to be learned here is not that roles and costumes are bad. In fact we can't avoid them—we play the roles of sons, consumers, lovers, givers, receivers, friends, children, young men, old men, allies, opponents, boyfriends, bosses, employees, worshipers . . . the list goes on and on and is in constant flux, even throughout the day. The problem is that, not armed with the truth about your self, your characters become both a means of survival and a means of suffering. The gay man who unconsciously believes he has no value unless he has a boyfriend learns to survive by creating boyfriends. But he does not heal the unconscious belief that he has no value. The character of "boyfriend" is there to help him learn that it is he himself who gives himself a sense of value when with a boyfriend and withdraws it when without.

The way out of belief in characters you've played that cause you pain or cover up your pain is to not confuse your true self with them, but rather to realize that all of your characters—both the ones you love and the ones you don't—are your creations. In this state of awareness you will not confuse yourself with any of your roles, but rather you will be able to acknowledge them as such. You will get the sense that the real you is not just the authentic individual behind them but the life force that animates the characters.

Why is this important? Well, to begin with, every role you play is a temporary one. Many roles you've played your whole life, like that of "son," for example, will end one day or maybe have already ended. Even that of "gay" and "man" will dissolve when your body dies. By this very fact, attachment to characters results in pain. Believe me, even attachment to "big-dicked hunk," no matter how much you worship yourself for it, is eventually going to come around as loss. That's because even big-dicked hunks don't last because perfect bodies don't last.

Just as important is the fact that it's hard to relate to others with love or authenticity when you believe you are your character. Rather, your attention is sucked into keeping it alive and proving its truths, and other people become in large part just a projector screen.

In recognizing all of this, the same decision is put to you as a "gay" male character that was put to you as a "straight" male character, which is to continue on in a state of passivity and unconsciousness—plugged into the Matrix, as it were—or to replace that passivity with a state of conscious living that recognizes that being able to play both "straight" and "gay" roles is a gift to help you see that all these differences are mirages, and to use this gift to help you realize the authentic, limitless, infinite self that is playing them.

Though this is hard work, the rewards of releasing the power you've given them over you are enormous. You've always had tremendous power; you just didn't realize it. By detaching yourself from identification with your characters you will realize, as I have, that they did not happen to you, but rather you created them. In seeing this you will be able to *consciously* access your infinite creative power, and thus come out of the finite realm of the "real" and into the infinite realm of the real.

Which Roles Have You Cast Yourself In?

When it comes to describing my particular journey and the characters I have played, in no way do I mean to imply that it is the same for everyone. Maybe you grew up in the projects in Detroit and totally identified with straight guys on the basketball court. Maybe you came into gay life as a teenage drag queen in Lafayette, Louisiana, and that's been your life for as far back as you can remember. Each person reading this, no matter how much he relates to the specifics of my life, has his own story line and plot points unique to him, and each has been the star of his own movie.

Regardless of the specifics of your journey up until now, the point of this chapter is to help you begin recognizing the characters you play, and the degree to which you believe you *are* these roles. There probably are many. As many gay men will attest to, it is an ironic truth about gay culture that as much as it has earned a reputation for freedom of expression, it is draconian in its demands that you identify yourself as a known character and that you stick to that script. Add to that the characters that straight culture imposes on gay men and most of us are left with very little range.

The first step toward freeing yourself of artificial limits is to become aware through *observing* the gay roles you play or have played, just so you can start becoming conscious of them as such. They could be based in ethnicity, like "gay black man," "gay Latino," "gay white man" or "gay Asian Pacific Islander." They could be sexual in nature, such as "top," "bottom" or "leather daddy." I even know a lot of guys who identify as "slut." They might be gender specific, such as "straight acting" or "femme-y," or they could be related to status, age or social construct, like "older gay man," "rich gay man" or "drag queen." You may tell yourself that you are an "outcast" from gay culture who does not belong and who is on the outside looking in, and that is a character, too. And they can work in any combination—a friend's boyfriend calls himself a "straight-acting white boy butch bottom." Whatever they are, the point is to identify the roles you play in order to bring them to the forefront of your consciousness.

Once you've started to get a grip on the various gay characters you play, start observing when you step into them and when you step out of them. For instance, if you create a profile on a sex or dating Web site, observe your power and intention to create a specific character and your will to make others and yourself believe that you are him. Or if you are threatened by another gay Latino who doesn't behave like you think a perfect gay Latin man should, that's a good time to observe your ideas of yourself that form a particular gay Latino character you are playing that are reflected in the other guy's choices. Get used to the idea that each one is indeed a role and that you are about to step into a play. That will help you to not only identify each role, but to also observe your creation of it from deep within your own being.

So ask yourself what roles you play. Write them down or just take notice when you see yourself stepping into one, whether it's "rejected ex-boyfriend," "porn star," "the guy nobody wants," whatever. Then begin to think about the characteristics of each one. In doing so you will shed light on a vast space inside of your mind that you are not usually conscious of but that is determining a great deal of your life for you.

Are You Playing a Character, or Is It Playing You?

In the vast space in your mind you will find an encyclopedia's worth of limits and demands and beliefs about who you should be and how you should spend your energy. The first of these is the idea that fulfilling the "reality" of a character is going to get you what you want.

Bring this idea to the surface and begin asking yourself what it is that a particular character is going to do for you. Ask yourself if you have experienced lasting happiness and fulfillment in your life through these characters, or simply highs and lows based on the success of your character. In other words, if you work yourself to death to maintain that you are a "masculine" gay man because you have a belief that your idea of masculinity is perfect and anything else is imperfect, then if someone says that he knew you were gay the second he saw you your entire sense of self might crack into a thousand pieces.

If your sense of self is so easily threatened, is it worth identifying with the character? And if it can be threatened, then is it real, or is it "real"? After all, if something is real it doesn't need you to defend it—but if it's "real," it dies without your defense. If your character would die without your belief in it, then take heart that it was never real in the first place, and you would lose nothing, and in fact gain everything, by detaching yourself from your identification with it.

This is especially true for any characters that you play that are victims of outside forces. For example, I was fooling around a few years ago with a guy who used to complain bitterly about people objectifying him when he stood behind the bar with his shirt off and his rump sticking out of his pants. And he would begin every sentence with "They think they can just objectify me."

But whose thoughts was he hearing? Whose "objectification" did he feel? Who placed him in that role? The fact was that he objectified himself, transferred it onto other people, and then complained about the fact that no one wanted to truly know him, thus in one swoop keeping it "real" to him yet letting himself not be responsible for the fact that he was the one who did not want people to know who he was behind the superstar bartender facade because he didn't know who he really was.

So try out noticing every time you hear yourself say, "He thinks this," or "She thinks that." For instance, with one close friend of mine who is very opposed to anything "feminine," I regularly find myself thinking, "He thinks I'm too feminine," and I feel victimized by him. Then I catch myself—who the hell is thinking this? I'm thinking this! Then I switch it to, "I think I'm too feminine." Try the same thing out, then make the thoughts grammatically correct by saying, "I think this," or "I think that." You'll not only heal yourself of victimhood, you'll find out what your character's real limits and self-judgments are all about. And outside of them, freedom.

Who Are You Behind the Scenes?

It is the fear of anyone seeing the "real you" that fuels such a deep identification with your characters. But chances are you don't know the real you. So it could very well be that your idea of the "real you" is in fact just another character you play, only you don't like this one. So if underneath your "fabulous" gay character that is perfect there is another character who believes he's totally unfabulous, pull that character to the surface, too, and expose him to the light of your awareness. After all, he's not real either and you do not have to believe in him anymore—he, too, is just a bundle of abusive ideas that go up in a poof once you've really looked at the truth of his existence. And he will never make you uncomfortable once you see him for who he really is.

Through observing all these characters you will discover what is real in you because what is real *is* the observer of all of them, and it is beautiful and perfect. Rejecting it is what makes you feel the opposite. This is especially poignant if you, like so many, are rejecting your natural loves and talents because they do not fit in with your character's idea of perfection.

For instance, my friend who is very upset by femininity went to an all-boys school and is so terrified of making any movements that might appear feminine that he is practically a robot. And he's very upset by people who talk with their hands (like I do!) because his "nongay-acting" character has judged it so despicably wrong. Nevertheless if he ever gets moved enough by something—like when his beloved dog does something really cute—he practically jumps out of his own skin, screeching like a child and flailing his whole body. And it is so natural and beautiful and adorable when this happens. That's when his "straight-acting" character's rejection of his natural way of expressing himself reveals itself, because at the heart of it is a decision to deny himself joy because he is afraid of looking "gay."

The point is that in identifying with a character you unconsciously reject who you really are. That sense of rejection is the only real rejection there is—there is no other—and it hurts. The fulfillment and sense of perfection that you desire can in fact only be realized through connecting to the you that animates the characters. This is where your true heart's desires exist. This is where the love song of your life plays. Listen to it and you will be happy. Listen to the robotic programming of your gay characters telling you that if you don't do the party drugs you won't be accepted or that if you aren't on the endless hunt for Mr. Right you will be cast out into the void and you will have a schizophrenic crack-up.

Which outcome do you want? This is a very important question to ask yourself because whatever the answer is is exactly the outcome you'll get.

How Attached Are You?

Looking next at how attached you are will reveal how strongly you believe that you yourself are the characters that you play. Exactly *how* attached you are can be observed many ways.

For instance, look for how much energy goes into maintaining your characters. Thoughts such as, "I *must* go to the gym no matter what," or "I *must* get that guy at all costs," are typical symptoms of extreme attachment because underlying these passions are fears of what it will mean to the life of your character if you don't fulfill them. Also observe fears you have that your life or an aspect of your life would be empty without being able to play a certain character, and how much it stings when other people do not reinforce a character you love or when they seem to bring to light a character you hate.

Bring these fears to the surface and consciously let them go in order to begin to create your life experiences without the fear. I cannot describe fearlessness to you, but trust me, it is amazing, and you will only find this out for yourself if you give it a try. If that means choosing to go out one night and *not* hunting for a guy, feeling the fear that arises, then letting it go and seeing that nothing bad happens—do that. It can be a very powerful exercise, especially if you find that in not being on the hunt you have the ability to pay loving attention to everyone who is in front of you just as you wish people would do for you.

Another symptom is rigidity. This can be observed when you are still acting out a role whose time has come and gone, such as in the emotional descent of a maturing gay man whose love for himself is completely contingent on his ability to look physically young. Rigidity also shows itself when you have unbelievably specific limitations on what you will allow yourself to experience, such as absolutes like I *don't* go to gay bars, or I *only* go to gay beaches. Shake those up by going places or speaking to people you normally block out—you'll find that your fear was a lot worse than what you actually find there.

Finally you can look for how much "us and them" and superiority and inferiority are in your character's worldview. The reality is that all humans are a shattered mirror of one whole unit, and each individual part contains the whole. Therefore no one could be better or worse than the other because each one *is* the whole. The fact is that everyone you see is simply a different aspect of you and what you see in them is yourself. Only your character could believe that you are inferior to someone who is younger or superior to someone who has less money. So get to know someone you think is inferior or superior and work through that illusion. Trust me, it is *very* healing.

Beneath your personal set of circumstances might also be a

number of unconscious beliefs about what it means to be gay that you have taken for reality, and limiting ideas about yourself that you have never questioned. Remember, being gay means nothing outside of what being gay means *to you*. Becoming aware of your beliefs in the same way you changed your ideas when you first acknowledged that you were gay will help bring a similar revelation.

Look for Limits on Masculinity and Femininity

You'll have to figure out for yourself what you believe you can and can't do and should and shouldn't do, but pay particular attention to limiting ideas of masculinity and femininity. Usually behind these ideas is a bunch of homophobic and misogynistic garbage. And trust me, if you are inflicting it on others, you inflict it on yourself, too. That's what "Judge not, lest ye be judged," from Jesus's Sermon on the Mount means: it's not that if you judge others that God or other people will judge you, but rather that what you judge wrong in others is simply a mirror of how you judge yourself. So it's not so much a commandment as a statement of fact that judging others is a symptom of self-judgment. When you stop judging yourself to be "wrong," you will naturally no longer judge others, but you have to begin with yourself. Anyway, you are what you are, and you like what you like—you don't need a gender qualification to make it real.

Look for Limits on Sex

If you tell people, "I *am* a top," or "I only sleep with people of a certain race," then you have taken your infinite sexual energy and squandered it on keeping a bunch of falsehoods about what is "perfect" and what is "not perfect" alive. *This is especially true if you unconsciously believe that how porn actors act on videos is how gay men should act in bed.* Asking yourself what taking on the role of a pornographic character can give you in the form of external power over another can transmute your experience from unconscious loss to conscious awakening.

Look for Limits on What Being Gay Means

You might have beliefs that being gay means that you must have or will have HIV, that you smoke crystal, that you are sexually insatiable, that you are inherently neater and more creative than straight men, that you will always be lonely, that you must have a boyfriend, or that you are less whole than straight people. Whatever your ideas about being gay mean beyond the gender you are sexually attracted to, trust that they are doing you no service at all. You are *so* much bigger than any idea that tells you that you must do or think or be anything because you are gay.

Look for Limits on Self-Love

Finally, this leads you down the road to realizing that at some point early in your life you made a decision that you would not love yourself if you did not meet certain expectations. Those expectations formed the characters you created in which you felt good to be yourself because you chose to love yourself in those situations. Choosing not to love yourself when you did not meet those expectations became the real experience of horror you have felt when you did not look like you were supposed to look, make as much money as you had decided you were supposed to make, or keep the boyfriend you had decided you wouldn't love yourself if you lost. You thought it was losing these things or these situations, but in reality it was choosing not to love yourself under certain conditions that caused the pain.

Letting Your Characters Go

The way out of these conditions and into freedom and awareness is to start paying attention to what your characters tell you, to question them, then to take away all the energy that you ever fed them. Don't feed them your faith, and they will die. Call the illusions out when you observe them. Acknowledge the tension and lack of happiness that results in staying committed to them. Allow roles whose time has come and gone to go. See the energy and intent from yourself that created them, and end the cycle altogether by no longer creating new ones—come into the present now, and you will find what true limitlessness is all about, and you will feel the love that you have denied yourself.

Of course, believing you are your character is not something that is unique to gay men—everyone does it—and the phenomenon is not limited to your "gay" characters. The same facts apply to every role you play.

In no way do I mean to imply that you don't have to go through what you have to go through. Repression never works because repression is about forcing something out of existence through denial and judgment. Going through what you need to do consciously and without judgment will allow you to see what is for what it is and then make conscious choices from there. That is the one key factor in making your gay experience a means to self-realization rather than just a route to another comatose way of living. And it is *never* too late. It is always a brand new moment, and the universe is eternally young. Any thought that it's too late in the game for you to change is indeed just the thought of your internal abuser trying to keep you in prison.

Once you have begun to live your experiences more consciously by putting these ideas into practice, and you begin to see that you aren't as rigid, that your life is opening up, that you laugh more, that you have so many more choices than you ever thought possible, that an abundance of wealth you didn't even know existed materializes before your very eyes, and that unexpected and delightful ways of expressing yourself seem to be coming out of nowhere, you'll know you're on your way. You'll find that being exposed for who you truly are is in fact a joy, and that exposing it to others is a joy, too. You will also discover that inspiration, answers, opportunities for fulfillment and means to happiness that you'd *never, ever even considered* are there for the taking just because you dropped everything else. Once you've really dropped your characters' story lines, you'll find that there was nothing to defend in the first place. And that's when you will realize that you had the power to put up the gates to Heaven, and you have the power to take them down.

4 Gay Men Are Not Dogs

Sex without reverence,
like business without reverence,
and politics without reverence,
and any activity done without reverence,
reflects the same thing: one soul
preying upon another weaker soul.

—Gary Zukav, *The Seat of the Soul*

The first time I sensed that my sex life had shifted into a place that I no longer understood and had no control over was in late summer of 1999. The day before I was to leave New York to spend a month working on a writing project in Provincetown with a photographer, I went to his East Village studio to pick up the laptop we were going to use. While the computer was being packed up, one of his assistants and I started cruising each other.

Every time we looked at one another I felt an overwhelming rush throughout my brain and body as if I were being injected with a drug. Within a few minutes we had introduced ourselves, felt each other up on the staircase, and made a date to "hang out" at my place later on that afternoon.

As soon as I got back home my whole life became reduced to hearing that phone ring. On the surface I figured this was a simple case of *want* (after all he was hot) and logic (I'd be stupid to turn down a hot guy); underneath there was conflict. Part of me absolutely wanted to go through with this; the other part was confused by the intensity of the rush and the speed of our encounter and wanted to slow down and get a grip on what I was feeling.

But I couldn't seem to step out of the situation and think clearly. It was as if the desire itself was controlling me, and I had no choice but to go through with it. And it wasn't exciting in the good way like when you anticipate something wonderful (which was how, up until that point, I usually felt about sex) but rather more akin to crashing from something and desperately wanting more of it to make you feel good again. You are very passionate about getting that something, but it's only in direct proportion to how bad the withdrawal is.

And I remained conflicted during our sexual escapade—part

of me was totally into it; the other part wanted to stop, but couldn't. I also felt different from how I usually felt during sex: instead of being aroused by intimacy, it seemed like it was "the scene" and the worship of each other that was the turn-on. Though the rush was powerful, there was an emptiness under-neath that revealed itself in full once the game was over, and I found myself feeling nothing for the guy whatsoever, and vice versa. Nor did I feel satisfied. In fact, after we were through all I was left with was the emptiness, and suddenly it was so potent that all I could think of was going out to pick up someone else in order to quell the withdrawal (which had now intensified).

Though I was vaguely aware of the anxiety, I did not look at any of this closely. Why would I? After all I was horny, I was attracted to him, and he was hot and into me. What's more, I had lived for twenty-four years with no men to sleep with at all, so if you thought I was going to deny myself you were crazy. Way in the back of my mind, too, was the thought that I had better get every guy like that while I was young enough *to* get them. And I couldn't think of a single gay guy I knew who wouldn't also have thought that turning this guy down was anything but insane or repressive.

I could not come up with one reason in the world why I should turn down an opportunity like that.

When I got to Provincetown, I found myself more and more *on the prowl* for sexual adventures like the one I'd just had. This was new for me—I had always worked a Marcia Brady hard-to-get image role. In fact, Marcia Brady had been my nickname among a lot of my friends because I always played it like it was the captain of the football team asking me to the prom or noth-ing. And there I was acting like a full-on sexual predator—or what I would later term a "marauder."

Becoming Sexually Lost

Confused as I was by this radical change in what I wanted sexually and how I was behaving, I still could not come up with a single reason—not even one—to not get every hot guy I saw if I could. And so I did.

On the one hand I felt free and unleashed; as if finally there was nothing stopping me. On the other hand I felt totally out of control, as if I had no choice in the matter. And I no longer felt satisfied at all—each encounter simply fueled the desire for another. Overwhelmed by the need to fill this insatiable black hole in me that kept growing bigger, I began to unconsciously allow all of my sexual energy to drain into it. I felt lost, with no idea where I was going or why, and out of control because I could not stop myself.

Over the next two years, I behaved as if I had been possessed by a powerful force. I was now almost exclusively venturing out only for sex; I never smiled at men I was sexually interested in anymore; I was suddenly interested in men who also looked like they were always on the make; and I became angry at men who did not cruise me back. From my perspective, my dark vibe became dark.

I found myself venturing out to bars and neighborhoods I would never have gone to before, where other men with dark vibes that resonated with mine went and where it was very easy to lie about who I was, often devoting hours and hours of a beautiful Sunday afternoon or a free Saturday night to finding the perfect sexual adventure. Even my long-standing tradition of rollerblading during the summer along the West Side Highway, listening to my Walkman and having a blast got sucked in and turned into nothing but another way to spend the entire day chasing after the perfect sexual prey.

And whereas in my sex life up until that point I had always been very intimate, gentle and passionate physically, I slowly lost all interest in physical intimacy. I just wanted to stand there, masturbate myself, and get off at the idea that I was hot, masculine, and powerful enough to get them off. And I wanted them to play it that way, too—that getting off with each other was something that two hot men do, and as I thought way, way, way, *way* back in the back of my mind, *it's not even really gay.*

The only conclusion I could come up with at the time was that I had just come into sexual reality—I thought that sex was never going to mean anything, so I might as well just go break it down, get what I wanted real quick, and get on with my life. But was being out of control what I truly wanted? That was reality? It didn't make any sense.

Despite the fact that I was so profoundly unconscious about it, I still knew to hide it. I didn't want people to think I was a typical sexually tragic gay man who was out of control and sleeping with men who were beneath him. I was above all that. And this was made easy by the fact I now only wanted to express myself sexually with men who did not exist in my social spheres; in other words, with men I did not respect.

In no way did this pornographic idea of myself I played resemble the rest of my life, so I kept strictly to a script of bullshit talk that simply negotiated the transaction. "What gym do you go to?" was intimate conversation for me. "Yo, wassup?" passed for introduction. Sometimes I would even lie about my name and my profession—"Tony the Trainer" was often my *nom de trick.* And yet part of the rush was the feeling that this was the *true me* finally getting a chance to let loose and be free.

Losing Sexual Control Altogether

Eventually the conflicted part of me was drowned out almost entirely. By the summer of 2001, I was fully consumed and blood thirsty, gorging like a perpetually starving stray dog psychologically incapable of a experiencing a full stomach. And I was cruising *all* the time. The world that I saw was a bar at 4 A.M. on a Saturday night. The streets were my "back room." How in the world had I gone all those years living in New York not realizing there were hot men available for sex everywhere all the time! And every time my phone rang I reacted like one of Pavlov's dogs. Which one is it—the dancer with dreads from the subway or the construction worker from Queens? "Oooooh yeah, it's an outer-borough area code—718! Must be the construction worker!"

If this had been bowel movements, we'd be talking about a diagnosis equivalent to life-threatening diarrhea, but I still could not come up with a reason to not pick up guys endlessly—the *need* in me was so pressing. The need was also insatiable and made it impossible for me to feel at peace.

This is not to say I did not have stopgap measures—I wouldn't put myself at serious risk for HIV, and I avoided the Internet, so I could at least have some peace in my apartment. But besides these limits, I let myself go. The fact is that not endangering myself in a tangible way actually enabled me because I felt I had nothing at risk.

And then, late that summer, I discovered what I had at risk when I suffered my first wake-up call: my erections went away. Suddenly, no matter how hot the guy or the scenario, I couldn't get excited, and I couldn't get it up. Talk about "shock and awe"; this got my attention.

At that point I knew I had two choices. I could up the ante by venturing into dangerous territory like unprotected sex or using crystal and Viagra in order to get excited again, or I could stop and take account of my sex life. Concluding that if I went any further I would lose my health and happiness forever I decided on the latter. Finally I had a reason not to pick up every guy I saw, or really any guy I saw.

So yet again I was forced to turn my attention inward. And I did so despite the fact that I knew on some level that looking at my sex life consciously was going to make my sexual fantasies disappear, which was the last thing I wanted. I thought if my fantasies disappeared, my sexual self would disappear, too.

Shining the Light on My Sexual Darkness

With my health and happiness on the line so that I was forced to examine my inner sexual life, the first insight I had was that I had not always existed in the sexual reality I had been in for the previous couple of years. In fact, over the course of my life, my sexual reality had changed substantially numerous times.

First I was in the closet for decades with no homosexual sex at all, so I was limited entirely to fantasizing about straight boys I knew. After I first came out I simply tested the waters—mainly, to find out if I was desirable, and to find out what and who I wanted. At that time just meeting someone and getting a number was mind-blowingly exciting because every aspect of the experience, even innocent flirting, was an enthralling mystery I was dying to solve.

Once I decided that there were men who were attracted to me, I went on to figure out who I was attracted to and who my fantasy men were. At that point I began seeking out beautiful, romantic figures (a glamorous trainer from South Beach was the crème de la crème to me) to prove I was beautiful and perfect like them. And if they took the bait, I would get my ultimate confirmation in the form of sex.

Even though that's what was really going on underneath, and on some level I knew it, I still loved the *idea* that we were being really intimate. And the way I was in bed reflected that—it was always an all-nighter with me, and I always wanted to see them again.

Then when I was twenty-eight I met a guy named Dom, and I got my first hint of what good sex felt like. In bed with him, every inch of my skin was a pleasure point. My emotions were so intense and the pleasure was so overwhelming I was actually shocked out of my incessant thinking during sex (Does he like me? Does he think I'm beautiful? Am I doing okay?) and into the present. With Dom I was as authentic as I could possibly be at that stage of my life, and in bed it felt like my whole being had opened up for him to gaze at. I felt as vulnerable and as loved as a baby, and my only concern was how much pleasure I could actually handle. I cried every time we had sex. Naturally I had no desire to have sex with anyone else, because no one else was Dom.

Then after only a few months he broke up with me and, in my mind, took that beautiful treasure away. At the time I told myself that there were lots of hot guys, and it was all the same, so it was fine.

But it was not fine. Examining my reaction for the first time three years later, I realized that I went into a severe state of denial because I couldn't cope with the rejection—and not just from Dom, but from every guy who had ever rejected me sexually. This was, in fact, a turning point in my sexual reality, because after Dom I did not create the same blissful experience, but rather I began to seek out men to control and to use, and whom I felt could take nothing away from me when we parted.

So my first realization was that my behavior had changed as the reality I created in my mind changed. Yet I was *still* desperate for my pickups.

Going Against the Grain by Questioning My Sex Life

Knowing that I was in a serious crisis, I began to seek out the advice of gay men I knew. Almost universally I was told that gay men are naturally promiscuous, and no different from straight men who would act like gay men if given the chance. What's more, it was made clear to me that to deny this "reality" through self-analysis, conscious awareness and discipline was sacrilege—that if I did not act out in these ways I was denying the essence of the reality of being a gay man. To question my sex life was repressive.

I was even more flabbergasted at the diagnosis, which was that my problems stemmed from the fact that I was thinking about it at all, because, as I was told again and again, *It's just sex, Chris. You're thinking too much!*

But I couldn't buy this. I'd crashed and burned at my physical peak, and I was miserable. There was no way I could accept that this was my destiny. So I decided to trust my instincts and turn my attention to my sex life—in spite of feeling like I was moving into unknown territory all by myself.

So I began work on my own to analyze every single desire I had and locate the unconscious thoughts and motivations behind my actions. I continued to feel what I was feeling, and desire what I desired, but this time *consciously*. I became partially functional again, enough to begin seeking out my cherished adventures once more, but this time around I observed myself.

The first thing I observed was that my fantasies were controlling my behavior. In other words, the *thoughts* were controlling *me*, not the other way around. So sexual reality wasn't "out there" on the streets and in the bars, it was my own head. In order to get control back I practiced recognizing my thoughts when they arose and then *letting them go*. This is when I truly began the process of sexual refraining.

Refraining is not the same as repression, so don't get them confused. Repression is trying to force something out of existence by denying that it exists or burying it so that it cannot be seen because it is "bad" or simply because you don't want to deal with it. It is not healthy, it is not conscious, it does not heal anything nor make anything go away, and it comes from a total lack of love because we only repress what we do not love.

Refraining is the process of stepping back from a certain reaction in order to observe it closely and see it for what it is so that it no longer has power over you. It has nothing to do with right or wrong, but rather with an intent to see what is actually going on inside you because you do love yourself.

Refraining is like stepping into an isolation tank—you're all alone with your thoughts, so you know it's you, not anyone else. Refraining from an unconscious reaction in this way is an express route from powerlessness to authentic power.

Sexually, this meant observing my reactions to my fantasies or to a hot guy and learning from them instead of automatically indulging them. In other words, I chose to refrain to the best of my ability from sexually marauding men for as long as it would take to clean up my mess. And if I did go through with anything, I studied myself intently by taking note of every aspect of the experience from beginning to end.

Refraining was fraught with anxiety for me because my consciousness was split—part of me was desperate to "go for it"; part of me knew the train wreck it would lead to, which was sexual diarrhea and impotence. Because the bigger part of me wanted to avoid the train wreck, I would stand right in the middle of my desperate hunger for a particular guy, and my absolute terror of not having sex, look at him and ponder: what is it that I am so insatiably hungry for? If it were sex I'd be satisfied by the sex, so it couldn't be sex. But that's what it felt like I wanted!

Discovering What I Was Really Hungry For

This was a *hideous* place to be. It was hell—I had all the pain and none of the anesthesia. But I stood there in the middle of this crisis, looked deeply into my being and forced myself to wake up. What I discovered as a result was that my insatiable desire wasn't for sex, but rather for a whole host of other things disguising themselves as sex.

What I was really hungry for was power over others to compensate for feelings of powerlessness in my life and to avoid ever feeling sexual rejection from anyone again. It was clear to me that men who were sexy and sexually "perfect" were very powerful—gay men *worshipped* sexually powerful men like they were gods. Becoming sexually powerful was the perfect way for me to live in the light of everyone's attention and acceptance, so I would never feel rejected or left out.

But it wasn't "everyone" who thought sexually powerful men were gods; it was me. I was the one who rejected myself for not being masculine or hot or good looking enough, and so I was the one who created a sexually powerful version of myself so that I would give myself that love and light.

The reason I was choosing men I thought were beneath me was so I could consume what I thought was perfect in them but not care if I was rejected. Only having sex with men I didn't respect also meant I wouldn't run the risk of showing who I am. So marauding was *exactly* what I was doing—which is to say, I was stealing from them what I desired (power, sex and attention) and taking from them what was missing in me (masculinity, acceptance and perfection).

Unconsciously I was also desperately trying to numb my growing fear of getting older and losing my sexual power, which I, years after feeling that first burst of power with the bar owner, did not know how I could live without. I was also compensating for a deep ocean of scarcity in my psyche when it came to sex—all those years of being a sexually constipated eunuch in the closet were spilling out now as sexual diarrhea. I was so terrified of being asexual again that I allayed that fear by gorging, and by indulging that fear to the nth degree I'd become impotent, which was the very thing I feared. Fear's goal is always to make itself real, and that's exactly what my fear had done.

And so I began to see why I had become insatiably hungry: I had equated sex with being powerful, accepted and free. Sex became morphine to heal the wounds underneath. But each time the painkiller wore off, I was desperate for another fix. I thought I was starving for sex because that's what all men are supposed to be like. But what I was really starving for was love and approval—not from anyone else, but from myself.

I Believed That Gay Men Were Dogs, Too

As I continued the excavation process, to my utter surprise I found a myriad of other factors controlling and creating my sexual "reality." I discovered that I, too, believed men were dogs, and so I was a dog, too. In fact I thought that being a dog *made* me a man, proved my virility and sex appeal, and that, in the end, that was all that I was, and there was no escape. And yet behind that was a contradictory belief that I'd find the ideal fantasy man this way, and if I wasn't endlessly seeking him out I'd never get him. I also discovered that pornography was in large part determining my behavior because I believed that what I saw in porn was perfect, and for me to be sexually perfect I needed to be like that.

As a fundamental function of this I unconsciously believed that the perfect sexual adventure would make me happy. After all, the sexual Nirvana sold in the gay male world indicated clearly that I'd be happy only if I could finally get the perfect guy. While it was clear that I was seeking out pleasure, in no way was happiness a function of my sex life. I was the opposite of happy—being horny in this state was for me full of anxiety, starvation and fear. I had, as the Dalai Lama speaks of, confused pleasure with happiness and was experiencing the destructive consequences.

Finally, underneath all of this was a searing judgment against myself for being what I considered a "typical gay man." The reason I hid my "typical" sex life from others was because I judged it to be wrong, which made me love myself, and every gay man I engaged with, that much less.

In short, my sex life was utterly without reverence, which is to say without respect or love for myself or for the men I wanted to get sex from. In the mythological sense of the human jour-ney, I'd found myself in the belly of the whale—swallowed up by my unconscious thoughts but believing I was still sailing freely on the ocean.

Knowing the truth because I was willing to look at it, I could no longer participate in my sex life as I had. It was time to heal my wounds instead of using sex as a drug to anesthetize them. It was the only way I could heal my addiction—and that's exactly what it had become, an addiction. It was also the only way I was ever going to get what I truly wanted, which was sexual fulfill-ment and to be at peace. In other words, I had no desire to be consumed by that whale, so I turned my full attention to becoming sexually conscious.

Healing My Sexual Wounds with Truth

The first change I had to incorporate was to love and accept myself for exactly where I was sexually. Realizing that I was deeply unconscious sexually did not mean I should judge myself for it, nor withhold happiness from myself until I changed. I had already silently judged myself to be pathetic and withheld love from myself as a result. Now it was time to embrace and love myself and realize that there was nothing, absolutely nothing, wrong with what I was going through sex-ually. It was simply a classroom where I was learning very valu-able lessons, and in fact I needed to love and revere myself for taking these lessons. After all, there could be no healing without love, so I needed to begin there by loving myself that very moment. It was not an easy task.

And in my sexual classroom, the first truth I had to accept was that I was the one who told myself that I was sexually imperfect. Having created this "reality," it was true to me. Trying to change this by proving I was perfect through sexual conquests would never heal me because I am not, in fact, more masculine, virile, powerful, accepted, hot or perfect by virtue of whom I can control sexually. I can convince myself for a minute that an activity or the opinion of another person can change my essence—which is exactly where the "morphine" feeling comes from when experiencing the illusion of external approval—but that sense then goes away when the external approval goes away, and I am left living again with the painful "reality" that I myself created.

So I began the healing process by working to release myself from my belief in all of these lies, in order to realize the truth about myself, which is that I am perfect just as I am. It is true I am not a model of traditional American masculinity, but that model is an illusion. And the truth about me sexually had been revealed to me in my experience with Dom: I had potential for sexual bliss and fulfillment, as does everyone, and it required no thought on my part whatsoever for it to exist.

The more I have released the fears about myself over the years, the more I have been able to avail myself of deeper truths about my sexual relationships. Namely, no man could reject me or take anything away from me. The hard truth was that I was the one who rejected myself. In doing so I unconsciously selected men who would "reject" me in order to physically manifest what was going on in my own mind so that my "reality" was "proved" true. That's why I never stayed sexually interested in someone who was available to me, and I did know, for example, that Dom was not completely available because he had recently been rejected by his boyfriend of many years and was distracted by getting his own acceptance back from that external source.

When Dom broke it off with me, my deep-seated fears that I was imperfect and sexually rejected were brought to the surface in a way that was too painful for me to accept. Because I was not conscious enough to recognize this and I did not have the skills or awareness to begin healing, I covered them up by becoming, in my mind, "sexually powerful." In doing so, I not only allowed my wounds to fester, I became addicted to the anesthesia, eventually losing my sexual power altogether. Recognizing all of this I was now making the choice to heal my wounds, though I also had a serious addiction to heal as well.

Learning How to Trust

Learning to trust did not mean that I needed to trust that no one would ever reject me sexually again. I did, however, need to trust myself that I would never make horrible and false deductions about myself and instead give myself the sense of acceptance and perfection that I was really after.

I could also trust that the universe would always supply exactly what I needed—my sense of sexual rejection and sexual scarcity was nothing but a fear. In such a state of peace and certainty I could show who I am authentically (good-bye Tony the Trainer!) and be profoundly vulnerable because no one, in fact, has power over me, and I have no power over anyone except myself. If I continued to love and accept myself, then that is what I would draw in sexually, and I would indeed stay fulfilled.

I was surprised to see that my sexual issues stemmed from intimacy issues, and I thought that was a cliché! I had to accept the fact that, as Tony the Trainer, the real reason I feared getting close in any way was because all those wounds of mine would get touched and I would recoil in pain.

Finally, I saw that outside of fear and pain there were millions of reasons not to pick up every guy I saw, the biggest of which was that I would never be sexually fulfilled that way. This is important to note because my unconscious sexual acting out wasn't just a misdirected attempt at happiness and an unconscious search for my own love and acceptance. It also represented an unacknowledged but deep-seated desire for sexual freedom.

Redefining Sexual Freedom

Some of my earliest memories are sexual ones. Around the time I was ten, I would walk into the woods behind the house and, when I felt I was far enough away from any sign of civilization that I could convince myself I was in the jungle, I would take off all my clothes and get very sexually excited while soaking up the feeling of being outside of time, space, family, society and restriction of any sort. And in my early teens, during the summer when I would often be home alone, I would walk around in the backyard in tight shorts when the garbage men would come around, and I'd feel the thrill of feeling sexually charged in front of men who were utterly outside of the world that I knew and therefore felt safe.

What these early expressions of my nascent sexual self reveal to me is that I was yearning to be sexually free at a very young age. One only yearns for freedom when one is imprisoned, and from my perspective there were two powerful prison guards I had to deal with—religion and homophobia.

Leashing Sex in Fear

Mainstream suburban Protestantism repressed sexuality of all sorts and kept it a dirty secret. Though of course this isn't exclusive to Protestantism—I don't know anyone who grew up anywhere in the world who did not absorb the notion that sex is bad, dirty and needs to be hidden. Even a good friend of mine who grew up in the sexually enlightened world of Amsterdam was taught that sex was naughty—which is why I believe he's so into bondage!

The second force that imprisoned me was a fierce suppression of homosexuality. In my mind, I couldn't reveal my sexual nature to anyone, so the whole flow of my sexual force was clogged, and I was seeking to let off steam in any way I felt I could get away with, hence my excursions to the "wilds" of my backyard and my adolescent peep shows I'd do for the trash guys from the other side of the tracks. Again, even friends of mine who were practically promiscuous with other boys going as far back as elementary school knew their homosexual activity had to be hidden and could never be acknowledged because of the ostracism that would befall them if ever labeled "gay."

But this prison of fear was only real to me because I believed in it. And I was in a great deal of pain as a result.

Rebelling Against the Leash

Coming out of the closet and entering into my sexual adolescence at the age of twenty-four was a profoundly liberating act against the fear. And the first few years were a genuine exploration of what I needed to go through to free up my sexual force. But instead of eventually moving beyond my reaction against repression and fear, I wound up becoming entrenched in it.

Thus I stepped into another prison, which was gay society's

map to sexual freedom, which is not authentic freedom—it is the *ego's idea* of sexual freedom. And the ego's idea of anything always starts with fear.

The gay world's map to sexual freedom does not actually lead to freedom because it is almost totally founded in reaction to the leash—in other words, in reaction to sexual repression and the judgment of sex, especially gay sex, as wrong and bad. When you act in reaction to pain and suppression, you don't free yourself of them. The only difference is that now you have sex to anesthetize yourself. The ego, which is to say the part of you that lives in fear, keeps itself alive through an endless cycle of pain creation and pain anesthetizing, or what I call the pain-morphine dynamic. It is a trap if there ever was one, because each feeds the other and in doing so keeps you forever from evolving because you believe that the trap is all there is.

Realizing There Is No Leash

But is the trap all there is? If you were to see that you still feel repressed sexually, and that underneath it all you are sure that gay sex is bad, you might see that, no matter how many men you sleep with, you are still chained to that leash. If on the other hand you chose to let go of the fear of being repressed and decided to release yourself of the judgment upon gay sex as "bad" and "wrong," you would find freedom from the leash altogether. You would escape the trap.

Sexual Healing Through Love and Acceptance

In addition to sexual freedom being equated with reacting to the leash, there is another aspect to the prevailing idea of sexual freedom that is equally erroneous, and it is that liberation comes in realizing that sex and love are two different things. A close examination of this reveals a much more complex picture.

The fact is that self-love and acceptance are needed to heal pain. Love is what ends the need for the morphine—and believe me, morphine is a poor substitute for love. If you think you've become liberated by realizing sex and love are two different things it might very well be that love is exactly what you're look-ing for from sex. You don't realize it because *it's not someone else's love you seek, but your own.*

The unconscious equation is usually something like this: sexual approval = love and acceptance. Doing without sexual approval is like doing without love and acceptance. That is like living without air. That creates a desperate need for sex or sexual attraction (though often it also manifests as desperation for a boyfriend or husband), which is really a desperation for the love and acceptance you are not giving yourself. The only way to feel like you are not asphyxiating is to have sex or to get a boyfriend. Once you get it, you feel relief from the pain for a period of time (this can also manifest itself in taking pleasure in degradation), but when your wounds are exposed again you find yourself back to living without air. So what is often called being a "horny gay man" or even a "lonely gay man" is often just a gay man des-perate for his own love.

This is the hidden reality behind the insatiable need for sex and what is generally perceived as "sexual freedom" in the gay world. A close friend of mine who was abused by his parents rather than loved and nurtured lives in insatiable hunger for sex, which he writes off by labeling himself a "slut" who is free to act in any way he pleases—even though he confesses that he rarely has any choice in the matter. And the sex stopped satisfying him years and years ago. Unfortunately the terrible pain and lack of love that sits in his being like a cancer is too great for him to feel, so every time it rises to the surface, it's time to go pick up someone. The pain does not come from not having sex; rather, it's the pain that is already there that is revealed when the anesthesia from the sex wears off.

This was absolutely true for me, which is why the more I healed myself, the less intense was my *need* to have sex to feel okay, which meant that I felt good whether I had sex or not.

The best example I know of someone else who realized this is my friend Ariel. He is gorgeous, young and sexy, and the fact that he picked up five or six men a week only confirmed the prevailing notion that he really had it made sexually. But when he finally began to question his sex life he confessed to me not only that he had been out of control for years, but that he lived in such terror around it that often he would collapse to the floor in tears when a guy didn't call back. Of course, no one knew this because he hid it.

With the help of a good therapist, he discovered that in growing up on a commune almost entirely removed from his parents he was suffering from a belief that his parents spent so little time with him because he was insignificant. Transferring that onto the boys in his commune and then onto gay men in New York, he became insatiably hungry for what seemed like sex, but it was, in fact, his sense that he mattered.

Stripping away the sex and waking up from the trauma of his childhood he learned how to stop telling himself that he didn't matter and that every time a guy didn't call it proved that he was insignificant. It was a difficult habit to break. But in the process he not only stopped suffering under the reign of this terrible idea, he healed a sex addiction that made mine look like child's play. It required him being brave enough to turn inward and face his horrific fears that he was invisible and mattered to no one, and that without the sex, he had to actually feel. Not to mention being brave enough to blow up his own spot by telling everyone the truth.

Removing Fear from Your Sexual Equation

The way to authentic sexual freedom is the way to all freedom: it lies outside of the ego, which is to say, *outside of fear.* This is an important point, because in the universe in which we live, there are only two emotions: love and fear. Every emotion and follow-through action comes from one of the two. From love, for instance, comes compassion, affection, selflessness, beauty, gentleness, clarity, intimacy, fulfillment, peace, bliss and awareness. Fear on the other hand masks itself with aggression, violence, insatiable hunger, conflict, confusion, anger, distrust, selfishness, anxiety and darkness. The ego, our finite idea of ourselves, is nothing but a ball of fear that co-opts valuable things (and sex is very valuable), while the infinite, true self is love, through which everything, including sex, can be channeled.

The good news is that love and all of its faces do not have to be created, so they do not need to be forced into your sex life, they only have to be revealed. The way to reveal the love, beauty, presence and transcendental potential in your sex life is simply to clear yourself up of all of the negative, fear-based emotions and beliefs that obstruct authentic sexual freedom and let the love inside of you flow.

In other words, you have to love and accept yourself completely in order to have a sex life that is without conflict, that does not masquerade as something else, that is no longer about seeking morphine for your pain, that is without underlying emptiness, that shows reverence for yourself and for your partners, and that gives you the sense of fulfillment and freedom that you truly desire.

We can only give what we have. If you have love, that's what you give, but if you live in loss, then you will project loss and seek only to take. The only way to change your behavior and get what you actually want from your sex life is to change your thoughts about yourself. In other words, you must get on the road to realizing who you actually are.

The ego's fear is that this revelation will neuter and emasculate the sexual self, because the ego knows nothing of what lies beyond it and is afraid of what's there. I am not suggesting, as the ego would have us believe, that to be enlightened is to no longer be sexual. Quite the opposite. I'm suggesting that to experience the true and pure nature of sex one must become enlightened, which just means to be aware and in acceptance of exactly who you are sexually.

Free Yourself from the Cult of Gay Male Sexual Reality

To become sexually aware you have to deconstruct what makes up your unconscious ideas about sex and your sex life. To understand your own sexuality it might be helpful to look at the pillars of gay culture's sexual "reality."

Gay male culture's idea of sexual reality is neither good nor bad, but it is a cult. And it is simply a mirror of mainstream society's cult belief that all men everywhere are wild tomcats who, without the neutering influence of women and marriage, would prowl and fuck and fight until they died. This is extremely destructive programming for it compels men to behave that way because they think if they don't, they are not men. Gay men suffer from exactly the same bad ideas, only we can never prove our manhood because of our fatal flaw in the form of whom we fuck.

So it is not a biological drive that compels men to act like dogs—it is the cult in control of our minds that needs us to believe in it in order for it to survive. As Don Miguel Ruiz says so poignantly in *The Mastery of Love*, we're talking about a hunger of the mind, not the body.

The gay male sexual cult is driven by many of the same forces at play in heterosexual life—fear of aging, of powerlessness, of vulnerability, of exposure and of love. This is why for many people one of the most "unsexy" things you can do is to show who you truly are, and this is why sex and dating sites are full of men crafting images they think will sell that bear little or no resemblance to their true selves, and why men are no longer hot to each other as soon as the fantasy fades and the reality of the complex being before them sets in.

This is also the source of the obsession with body parts, sexual roles and fetishes. Though the cult needs you to believe this, there is no such thing as "just sex." There is always added meaning that makes sex desirable. So without the added meaning of love and intimacy, you need the added meaning you associate with a gigantic this, a shaved that, a particular "scene" you're currently into or someone who playacts a certain role. That's because a body on its own is not enough. That's why you can have two people who look virtually the same, yet one turns you on and the other does nothing for you.

This is not to say that role-playing and fetishizing aren't real sex—getting turned on by the added meaning of acceptance and perfection unconsciously ascribed to a prop is indeed sexual energy. It is, however, an unconscious energy, one that looks like one thing but is something else entirely, which is the very nature of unconsciousness. There is no reason to judge it or yourself, either—it is what it is. But that is the point—to see it for what it is, not how it appears, because that is the way out of the cult and into freedom.

Sex as an Expression of Pain

Role-playing is no doubt the dominant sexual frequency in gay society today. We don't want to show who we are because we hurt underneath. We unconsciously believe that that pain *is* who we truly are because we know we do not match up to our ideas of perfection. Nobody does, but we do not see this because we live in a state of projection—it seems as if it's other people who reject us. Naturally, then, we wouldn't want genuine intimacy during sex because closeness hurts—it gets us too close to feeling the pain and weakness that's underneath, and that is anything but sexy.

But if you realize those wounds are not you and that they can be healed, you will want to be close because it will feel good, and in that state you will tune in to a higher frequency of love, selflessness and intimacy in your personal relationships. Your sex life will then naturally reflect this desire, and you will no longer try to fulfill your need for intimacy (and you do have a need for it) with purely physical closeness that is actually a big distraction from the fact that you and your partner aren't close at all.

A lot of gay men know this from experience. A close friend of mine admits he always thinks he's "in love" with the newest guy he's met at a club or the gym—that is, until he's had his way with him. At that moment, his fascination turns instantly to disgust, and unwilling to tell him that he's no longer interested, he turns on his computer and stares at the screen, ignoring his guest until he gets the picture. When his computer makes its start-up sounds, it's like a gong going off in his apartment that says what he's really feeling, which is "get out!"

It may seem that his fascination for the guy turned into disgust, but the truth is that the disgust was already present and is simply revealed once the spell is broken. And the harder truth is that it's not disgust for the other guy—it's disgust for himself. Sex in this way can be all smoke and mirrors, and it takes a lot of attention to begin to see what's really going on.

Once you begin to heal your pain and feel more of your own love, the fact that you do not actually care about the other person in a low-frequency sexual vibe will become painfully obvious to you. It will also be intolerable, because a lack of love and respect is by its nature quite painful because it is only our own that we feel.

Even if, as with me, your sexual instincts sometimes still direct you to an unconscious encounter, as you heal within your current sexual reality you find that you can never be cruel and unloving, even after the fantasy has disappeared. I'm always loving to men I feel unconscious sexual vibes with because it is my own love that I feel, and in showing it to them I love myself in return. In accepting them I accept myself. I elevate what was meaningless into meaning. Believe me, it feels a lot better than disgust!

The underlying feeling of emptiness and disgust at oneself is why some men willfully risk contracting HIV through unprotected sex—the pain is so great that they'll do anything to cover it up right now. This is the trap of the pain-morphine dynamic at its most destructive, because this type of sex results in considerably more pain, which creates that much more need for anesthesia. The only thing that can cure that trap is love.

The Need to Be Close Is Real

Of course closeness is a big part of this equation because the need to be close is real. It reflects the only reality there is, which is complete oneness. When you look at it this way gay men no longer appear like a bunch of rabid dogs off the leash, but like a bunch of human spirits desperate to feel their own love and to connect deeply with others in order to realize who they truly are. The current method may actually produce the opposite result, but the desire to be close is as right as rain.

Find Out If You're Ready
to Examine Your Sex Life

Often, the will to question your sexual reality only comes to those who finally accept that they aren't feeling any of the things they want to feel. But I do not presume everyone has the same experiences. The route and the behavior aren't where revelation lies—negative and fear-based emotions can play themselves out in every sexual scenario. There are gay men who are monogamous but who simply project their fear-based sexual selves on one partner, very promiscuous gay men who unconsciously believe they will "find love" at the bathhouse, gay men who hide from their unconscious sexual selves in sexless lives, and physically monogamous gay men who spend their days daydreaming about sex parties.

But making a change is not about forcing a change in your behavior. My friend Mark who says he can't go to a gay bar and not pick someone up has been trying for years to force himself to change because he doesn't like the fact that he's not in control. But until he's ready to find out what it is that he's truly looking for, his desires will not change. Examining the unconscious thoughts behind his behavior is what is necessary to discover freedom.

In my conversations with gay men on this topic, I have found there to be a great deal of defensiveness of the prevailing ideas of sexual freedom. You may also believe that what you've experienced up until now is all there is, so you know how men are, and that's that. These defenses can make self-analysis very difficult. The other problem is that once people stop covering up their pain with sex then they feel their pain, so the suggestion that you stop covering it up is tantamount to telling you to be in pain. Adding all this up you really have to be ready to heal at all costs—including letting go of your beliefs and feeling pain that you have been running from—in order to set forth on a different path. But when this destiny, no matter how hard it may be at first, seems more desirable than your present, you'll know you're ready to finally figure out what truly ails you, and how it can be healed forever.

Heal Your Sexual Self

All healing starts with a release from fear. But you can only start to heal if you are aware of parts of you that are in need of healing. Becoming conscious is healing because nobody would *consciously* injure themselves or others physically or psychically. But the very nature of *unconscious* behavior makes it difficult to get a grip on because you aren't aware of it.

It helps to understand that in our lives there are different frequencies that we tune in to with each other. If we have fear and self-rejection inside us and avoid knowing ourselves, we are turned on by people in the same state. If we have love and acceptance and are getting to know who we truly are, then we are hot for people with those same qualities. That's the way it goes. It can't be helped.

In a state of sexual unconsciousness you can't see this. That's why it was only after I cleaned myself up that I could see what was written all over the faces of all the men I was hot for no matter how "masculine" or powerful they seemed, which was loss and need. This reflected me perfectly.

But it's very easy to not see how our partners reflect us. A close friend who is a rich and successful celebrity hairstylist gave up years ago trying to make something satisfying for himself sexually because he said he finally accepted that he couldn't help being sexually attracted to street hookers. I understood where he was coming from entirely. But what was missing in his puzzle was the realization that just because he was a rich stylist and they were poor street hookers didn't mean that they weren't remarkably similar—in his partner's lack of self-respect and need to have power over others and over other men he has the opportunity to see himself. Blinded by the externals, he can't see that they mirror him, and in ignoring this he ignores the lessons in the faces of his partners that could help him get what he readily admits he truly wants, an intimate relationship with someone he loves.

In practicing looking at whom I am attracted to as a mirror, my sexual frequency has changed dramatically. Now that I am no longer in a gigantic state of loss and need, I'm not hungry to feed off men who seem to be living in loss. But it did not require me to force a change. In fact you cannot force a change in who you are sexually attracted to nor what you want to do sexually, but you can tune in to a higher state of consciousness, and when you do, your sexual reality will naturally ascend, too.

But you have to work where you are at any given time. Every time I introduce compassion into an otherwise unconscious sexual transaction I make a conscious shift out of fear and into love in the very moment that love is needed most. It's true I've given up a lot of "hot scenes" as a result—it's true you can't really buy into the fantasy anymore once you know what's going on behind the scenes—but in being brave enough to drop the act and show who I really am, I'm turning the page sexually and evolving into a whole new being.

Changing Your Sexual Frequency

To change the frequency you're resonating on requires work. Before, you saw things for how they seemed—I'm horny—and now you look for what might be behind it—I'm in pain. You have to let go of the "horny" morphine in order to feel what is giving you pain underneath. It goes against everything you've been taught about sexual freedom, but most of what you've been taught about sexual freedom is not true.

This means questioning all kinds of things you've never questioned before. The test of whether something is real or not is whether it still exists when you stop thinking it, so there's a risk you might find that your sexual "reality," in fact, doesn't exist. If you think that playing the role of a guy who can get anyone he wants will make you happy, and you realize that you are not happy in that role, then you are faced with letting go of what used to be a pillar of your sex life. If like my friend Ariel you find that pretending to be a ghetto thug isn't doing it for you any-more, you have to let go of that fantasy, even if you've never known sex outside of playing that role. It's scary, but the poten-tial is there for you to learn to consciously create what you wanted in the first place, which is fulfillment.

The good news is that anything, and I mean anything, includ-ing addiction, that is brought into the light of consciousness will be healed and transmuted. Your sex life is no different. Bringing the unconscious thoughts into awareness will introduce choice and thereby dissolve addiction. But you cannot make accurate choices until you see things for what they actually are. Doing so requires the work of unveiling.

Look at What's Going On Behind the Scenes of Your Sexual Play

To begin, take a look at what is going on in your mind by doing some self-examination.

Look at your sexual attraction to external power. The baseline defense is that "power is hot." But desire to use sex in order to have "power" over others is simply fear with a mask. So look behind your desire to have power over your sexual part-ners or for your partners to have power over you and you will find fear—of being used, of showing your love, of being who you truly are, of being vulnerable and a host of other expres-sions of your real self. When you begin to see expressions of power as expressions of fear and weakness, it's not quite so hot any more.

See the connection between pain and sex. Do this by watching to see if you find yourself seeking out sex when something painful happens or if you are in some sort of pain when not experiencing sexual arousal. This means flipping the picture from seeing not having sex as causing pain to seeing your existing pain exposed when not having sex.

Take a look at your fantasies. Like power, fantasy has taken its place as a definitive part of sex, especially as delivered through porn. Fantasy is often chalked up as biological sexual arousal when, in fact, it is usually the fantasy in your mind that generates the sexual excitement, not the other way around. But fantasies can be nothing but programmatic ideas keeping you from experiencing anything else. So rather than simply unconsciously indulging them, question them and find out what they mean to you and what enacting them means *about* you, and you will gain powerful insight into why you are the way you are. The other problem with sexual fantasies is that you and your partners simply become characters in them. Letting the fantasies go offers an opportunity to experience yourself and the self of your sexual partner in a considerably more authentic way.

Observe tendencies toward self-destruction, danger and degradation. If you are sexually aroused by humiliating or being humiliated by someone else, this is a symptom of self-contempt. Love for yourself will heal this, for there is no part of you that is not worth total love. You are love itself, but you must start with honesty to discover this.

Watch for how your frustrated need for genuine intimacy reveals itself. It is easy to be physically intimate, but because of our emotional pain and defenses it is difficult to be genuinely intimate. Therefore physical intimacy becomes a crutch for lack of genuine intimacy. But if you allow yourself genuine intimacy you will not need a crutch, and your sexual life will become an accurate reflection of your relationship and your real feelings about yourself and the other person, not a compensation for it.

Revisit what anonymous sex means to you. Anonymous sex is *never* "just sex" because the point of anonymous sex is that you can project your fantasies onto the person without any obstruction in the form of who they really are and who you really are. Even sex with a partner we love can be "anonymous sex" if we hide our real selves during sex. Repressing it or labeling it "wrong" is not the answer—looking at what it actually means to you, however, can be incredibly enlightening.

Compile all the fears that play out in your sex life. Fear of sexual scarcity is an often unacknowledged fear, and accumulating sex will never heal it. Letting go of the perception of scarcity through examining your unconscious beliefs will help you realize abundance. Similarly, using sex to cover up whatever fears you've got—of getting older, of being excluded, of not being loved, of not being attractive—will not make those fears go away. Seeing that those fears don't exist will.

Observe in a sexual transaction whether you are taking from your partner or loving him. Focusing on taking from the other person rather than loving him may be the standard frequency on which gay men are operating sexually, but it is not resulting in happiness. And the whole premise is fundamentally flawed because the unconscious belief is that the other person has something you need to get from him. But after you "get" him, the feeling of having replaced what is missing in you departs. That's because it's your own love that you seek. And I ask you, have you ever seen anyone on the hunt who looks happy? I never was. Switch from taking from the person to loving him, and you will discover the love and happiness that you were looking for all along.

To really get down to the nitty-gritty, record all of your sexual beliefs. You may believe that scoring men will *make* you virile, sleeping around with tons of men is the same thing as freedom, or that sex will *make* you happy or fulfilled. Put the beliefs to the test, and if they do not pass muster, let them go.

Tune into how much choice you feel you actually have. Any time you are seeking out sex even though part of you doesn't want to, you are being compelled by fear; an aware state of mind is never compelled by unconscious thoughts and beliefs. *A conscious mind has a choice—an unconscious mind does not.*

Look out for other inauthentic aspects of your sex life, such as: what you define as "normal" but might really just be an excuse to not examine yourself; qualities you look for in a partner that you think you lack, such as masculinity, beauty or success; and a desire to own what you find beautiful, desirable or sexy.

Instigating a Whole New Sexual Practice

Looking at all these dynamics can feel overwhelming. It can also seem that by removing all of these negative forces there'd be no sex life left to be had. That is because these fear-based dynamics have ingrained themselves with sex to the point that we've confused the pollutants with the substance that is polluted. Freedom is freedom from the single greatest pollutant in our sex lives, which is fear. Removing fear from your sex life is the way to sexual freedom.

Once you've observed these dynamics in play you can begin to change your external sexual reality by changing your internal reality. To do this requires having different practices from what you've had and from what is considered, for lack of a better term, "normal" in gay life. Ariel first started off by not kicking out his tricks as soon as he was done with them and being loving, honest and considerate with them instead. This was so meaningful because it was indicative of the fact that he was increasingly less disgusted by himself. Another guy I know who was addicted to jacking off with guys in the shower at the gym found himself one day compelled to bring over a fresh towel to his gym trick afterward, rather than bolting off the second he was done. He did not do this out of guilt, but out of love and respect. This is the type of spontaneous act of love for another that can only come out of loving yourself. As tiny as it may seem, it is a saintly act nonetheless because, like Ariel, he is learning to love himself and others in very difficult, unloving conditions. And as amazing as it is, and as brave as they are, there's no doubt about the fact that this kind of selfless, loving behavior is all very abnormal in the gay world.

But what is normal right now in gay life results in a lot of pain. So it's not helpful to you to use that as your base. Create your own base by being brave enough to realize that you are immensely powerful, and you don't need other people—especially other people who you see, when you look at their lives honestly, are not happy or fulfilled themselves—to tell you what to do or how to think.

Instead, do this: practice giving yourself the same feeling of love and acceptance that you get when a delicious guy gives you "the look," and you will discover what happiness and sexual freedom are all about. From there, sex will become all about sharing this abundance with someone else, and by the laws of nature, you will naturally attract someone else looking to share their abundance with you, too.

Go Sexually Where Few Gay Men Have Gone Before

There is no getting around the fact that it requires giving up immediate pleasure in order to heal deep unconscious fears and emotional wounds. It's a tough pill to swallow because it requires struggle and sacrifice in order to get there. In order to let something new in, you have to empty out. The emptying process feels exactly like that . . . empty. In this case, as you extract these elements from your sex life and see that they no longer exist, the first thing you feel is loss.

This doesn't mean that your whole sexual movie comes to a complete stop and you just sit there in desolation—it means that you continue to live out your sex life but this time around you do so *consciously*. Once you've let go of the unconscious ideas that sex equals acceptance, and you give yourself that acceptance all the time, you'll have no problem letting sexual opportunities with strangers go because you're giving yourself what you used to think you had to get from them. And without that motivation, you can easily let a hot guy just keep on walking, and miraculously, experience no sense of loss.

In this state when you do feel a conscious desire to get to know someone in all of their dimensions and to share all the dimensions of your own being in a real, intimate way, you'll know to stop and pay attention *because you will recognize the feeling as innately good and the attraction as deeply real.* And you'll be able to accept it because you are no longer averse to the nitty-gritty of someone's depth when you are not averse to your own.

Becoming conscious of my own sexual reality has been excruciating and frustrating, no doubt about it. With each stage of significant development, there is a death, then a resurrection, and I definitely continue to feel the death part. I'm no longer where I used to be, but not fully where I'm gonna be, and it's no fun, but that is the nature of transition.

I find that the struggle to show who I am and to be loving is worthwhile because even though I've given up tons of sex with lots of different guys, I've also given up the underlying emptiness that fed the need for it. In learning that I am already filled to the brim with everything I need, I'm on the path to learning how to share this sexually with someone. This is my intent. And it's a good intent to have because it comes out of reverence. And reverence feels amazing because reverence comes out of an innate sense that everything and everyone, including me, deserves respect and love. We are all a part of the one divine force, and nothing or no one is outside of it. And sex, absolutely, is divine.

It is also, for me, a profound act of liberation to learn how to use my body as a vehicle for love rather than a temple of power. Again this one is very tough. I was programmed to use my body for power, and it became my armor to hide how hurt I was and to allow me to take from people as I pleased. Being strong enough to drop that act has shown me that I'm so much stronger and more powerful than a tight T-shirt could ever have made me feel. Not that there's anything wrong with tight T-shirts—it's just that an addiction to the external power they give me doesn't get me what I actually want.

It's also amazing to have this choice, to feel certain about what I'm doing and why, to be on the path to getting what I want, to recognize I'm getting what I'm ready for, to not have a gaping hole in me that I'm futilely trying to fill through sex, and to be totally sane sexually. I'm here to tell you that *that* is sexual freedom because I am now conscious and in charge and healing. This involves zero repression because there's nothing to repress. Sexual freedom also means I can go rollerblading or even out to a bar and have fun again because I no longer have a black hole inside of me making me miserable, desperate, afraid and starving. And if those kinds of feelings show up, I do my best to heal them, then move on.

These days I can think of plenty of good reasons not to have sex with every guy I see, so it is now as easy to not pick up people as it is to not eat birthday cake at every meal or not start a fight with everyone who steps in front of me in line at the grocery store. I can also love myself for that part of me that is still where I used to be and not detach from it because I've judged it to be wrong. And this is the most crucial thing, because it's easy to turn awareness into another tool to hurt yourself with. But that is not true awareness; it is judgment against yourself with a mask. Loving yourself for exactly who you are sexually *right now* is true awareness.

With all these changes, it's like I've become something I didn't even think existed, which is sexually *wise*. And I can also tell you this: the wisdom I've gained from getting off the sexual merry-go-round is incomparably more valuable than what I could get from a million blow jobs from a million dream men. I'm not saying that you have to stop having sex for a period of time—or less sex than you're having now—that was my journey. What I am saying is that in bringing consciousness to your sexual inner life your behavior will naturally change because your reality is changing. Just be open to what change that may be. Trust that you're always going to get exactly what you're ready for sexually, and if there comes a time when you're ready to deal with scary stuff going on behind the scenes, then that's what you'll get. And if that happens and you see a lot of changes, it's time to celebrate because it means you're healing.

Though the focus of this book and this chapter is on *you* personally, not on "gay culture," it is glaringly obvious that many gay men are going through a serious trial but do not yet have awareness of it. The illusions of gay sexual reality *are* the trial. They are the belly of the whale.

The only way to get out of the belly is to realize that you are there and set an intent to get out. So the only thing that does matter is you. And what matters with you is thought, for that is where behavior comes from, and that is where all the potential for correction and evolution lies. By cleaning up yourself, by choosing to love and accept yourself unconditionally, by realizing that you are whole and missing nothing, and most important, by dropping the past and the future and coming into the present, you do your part in bringing light to the darkness of the gay male sexual world. Not in the goal of creating an illusory external sexual Nirvana, but in revealing an authentic personal Nirvana, and then in turn helping to liberate others. In the process we also get the sexual freedom—and the happiness—that we truly long for, and which we deserve.

♂ 5 Love Doesn't Hurt— Fear Hurts

You don't need anyone else to love you. Love comes from the inside.

—Don Miguel Ruiz, *The Mastery of Love*

For the majority of my life I have had a great deal of pain and drama in the relationships I have had and in the love that I felt. This was not the case for the first ten years. I had great relationships with my family, and fulfilling and uncomplicated friendships with my mom, my beloved cousin, Ashleigh, and my best friend, John Paul, in addition to feeling good and happy in my relations with school mates, neighbors and the like.

Then sometime around age nine or ten, right when I began to feel rejected and excluded by my peers, the way I experienced my life, the love I had in it and the relationships that filled it up began to radically change.

Though derision on the part of my childhood peers was intermittent, my own attack on myself became relentless and exhaustive. The more I realized that I was never going to be the straight, masculine guy on the football field with the girlfriend, the more I began to feel there was nothing right about me at all. I went from being ebullient and outgoing to depressed and withdrawn, and I spent much of my early adolescence in bed asleep trying to escape the nightmare of my waking life.

My relationships became utterly poisoned. Not only did I feel rejection emanating from people all around me, I also became so desperate for love and approval that even the slightest bit of positive attention could make me feel like I was in love. And often I thought I was!

In my early teens I began to extend my personal rejection outward by rejecting everything that I thought represented me that was not good enough. Our cars weren't expensive enough and our house wasn't big enough, but the nexus of this rejection was my father, who suffered from a debilitating form of schizophrenia that ruined his personality and laid waste to his intellect. He was filthy in his living habits and would hoard newspapers and junk of all kinds. I not only wound up spending my teens avoiding him and hiding him from people I knew, but also endlessly trying to erase evidence of his existence.

The primary way I did this was through cleaning and maintaining our house as the on-site maid, yardman and redecorator. I felt like I was on an endless quest to prevent the house from being overwhelmed by a tidal wave of crap that was going to wash over us if I was not eternally vigilant. And I was vigilant—often the first thing I would do when I got home from school was vacuum—because I was terrified not just of being overwhelmed by crap, but by what my father's crap meant about me.

Meanwhile, I managed to maintain a handful of wonderful relationships, namely with my mom, Ashleigh, and my best friends in high school, Robert and Mary Margaret, all of whom provided me with an envelope of unquestioning and nonjudgmental love and acceptance, and each of whom I had tremendous chemistry with. But I was so focused on trying to get approval from people I thought had rejected me that I did not realize that I *already* had perfect relationships.

As I mentioned earlier, my first big attempt to remedy my sense of rejection was a campaign to remarket myself with a new image. And I was very ambitious: I built myself up (the first place I drove with my new driver's license on my sixteenth birthday was to a gym), corrected my posture and my walk (I was pigeon-toed), cajoled my mom into buying me the perfect preppy wardrobe, got braces, and cleared up my acne with medication. Then I began to parrot how the popular boys talked and walked and set about repressing my feminine and flamboyant ways. When it comes to makeovers, much to my pleasure I discovered that I was a natural.

Unveiling the New Me

And things did change. After I left for college in Mississippi and began to experience all the popularity I had ever wanted and was free from even having to look at my father or the kids I grew up with, I patted myself on the back, looked back on all that baggage in Birmingham and thought I'd vanquished my enemies.

But there was a big glitch in my new matrix. I may have changed locations, but I carried all that baggage with me, and the symptoms were severe. I was extremely paranoid that all my friends were secretly rejecting me behind the scenes. Thus, I was constantly introducing a lot of drama in my relationships. I blamed, broke up, judged, pined, longed, and experienced har-rowing highs and tragic lows depending on who gave me what kind of attention when and why. I built up my friends when they conformed to my wishes and judged them unworthy or, con-versely, "fell in love" with them when they didn't. I was, in the collegiate dialect of the time, quite "psycho."

My relationships with men were particularly loaded. I still desperately longed to be and act like a "normal" guy, so my acceptance by males was a morphine fix that I was prioritizing higher than any of my treasured, loving, long-time relation-ships. I was so "in love" with my friend Andy, who was in every way the football player with the girlfriend, that I would have dropped any of my actual close friends to spend even a second with him. In my mind he really had "it," and if only I could be with Andy I could finally be happy and whole.

But I was gay and he was straight. I was feminine and com-plex and he was simple and masculine. I was flawed and he was perfect. Maybe I could be perfect if someone like Andy was gay and would want me and love me, too, but I believed that was never going to happen.

The New Me, Part II

I learned how to compensate for these feelings of inadequacy by becoming a social persecutor, and that was the level of consciousness I carried with me to New York. There I manifested a full-time job creating and mastering a world-class image of coolness and invincibility. The big difference was that in New York, I could be gay and perfect. So this time around I felt I really had my chance to *be* perfect.

Of course this was the time in my life when I could actually act on my crushes and infatuations with men. I could finally get my Andy, though now my Andy was a shirtless bartender from Sydney.

And when I scored him I was on the mountaintop because the successful score meant I was gorgeous and sexy, and I would wile away the hours replaying how he indicated that I was hot and perfect enough for him to want me. When I was rejected, I was back into the void, burning up with resentment and melting in depression, again feeling that I was gross and weird and being cheated out of my due.

As I moved into my thirties and became a blistering critic of gay men—they're so immature, they're so self-destructive, they're so slutty, they're so self-involved, they're so full of themselves—it became easier to remain safe from ever being hurt by a gay guy again. I couldn't stand to even look at them—that is, unless I found them sexually arousing.

This was also my solution to my conflicting ideas about relationships. On the one hand it was my firm conviction that relationships, straight or gay, were really just bogus and boring acts of infatuation, fantasy and weakness. I thought, "Look at all these tragic guys in their phony relationships. What losers!" On the other hand was my secret fear that the reason I never had boyfriends was because I wasn't good looking and sexy enough to play that role for someone. This caused me to resent gay men in a major way.

As I had my entire life, I still had very close and intimate relationships. Friendship is a natural talent for me that, unbelievably, even my life of insanities has never been able to totally squash. But by my early thirties I was focused entirely on people who did not "upset" me, which meant that almost all of my healthy relationships were with women. (And I thank God for the amazing women in my life because they showed me what healthy relationships are all about.)

After all, I did not trust gay men because they were so fucked up. In my mind even my closest gay male friends had done me wrong in one way or another—by not respecting me enough, by judging me, by behaving in self-destructive ways that made me angry, by disagreeing with me or by valuing other people (usually tricks and abusive boyfriends) more than they valued *my* precious friendship. When I shared my bedroom with my best gay friend so he could get on his feet financially, and I realized three months into it that he had not saved a dime, I decided that not only had I been used but that giving so selflessly would always mean that I would be used. So I kicked him out of my place and out of my life.

By keeping everyone who "upset" me at a distance, my life indeed became less emotionally dramatic and painful. I was then convinced that the drama of life was *out there* in people who were messed up and not together like me. All I had to do was keep everyone out who was upsetting, and it would all be fine.

Problem: solved.

And then Robert came into my life.

My Wounds Exposed

I met Robert when I was thirty-two by sexually marauding him on the street. But as soon as he opened his mouth the curtain closed on my intention to act out my sexual fantasies and opened up on something else entirely. As he told me about himself—he was a twenty-seven-year-old artist from the South who had just gotten out of a long relationship—I felt myself resonating in parts of my being I wasn't sure I had ever felt before. The resonation was so deep that it felt more like a recognition than an introduction. And I heard the silent voice of knowledge speak up—it told me that he was going to be a big, *big* part of my life.

But what we were to do with each other was not so obvious. At this time, I was still in the grips of compulsively marauding men on the street—after all, that was how I met Robert in the first place—but I wasn't able to act on it anymore. Similarly, Robert was still emotionally devoted to his ex-boyfriend and not ready or willing to have sex or get involved with anyone else.

We were both conflicted but we did wind up going on a date to get to know each other. And because I knew I wasn't really available, I was relaxed and wasn't even upset that he was still fixated on his ex-boyfriend and talked about him all the time. Another deluded romantic soul in need of de-programming, I thought.

As we got closer and closer over a very short period of time, we began to say that we were dating each other. I also began to feel my love for him really blossom in a big way. And that was when my attitude started to change: I began berating him when he would break dates with me to spend time with his ex, judging him for his obviously screwed-up attraction to a screwed-up guy (his ex-boyfriend was abusive), and withholding attention in order to get him worried that he was going to lose me. My state of fearlessness vanished, and I found myself terrified I was going to lose him. Ever so slowly the love, acceptance and selflessness I had been feeling was replaced with anger, paranoia and self-ishness. I stopped having fun and started being tense.

But those were just warning tremors. The volcano erupted when one time he left me waiting for him for hours without a call. When I finally spoke to him and found out he was fine, I exploded.

I decided right then and there I'd let an "upsetting" person in. He was clearly untrustworthy, so I needed to break up with him. He obviously didn't give a shit. He was obviously a liar. God, was I wrong to trust Robert!

So I blasted him for being selfish and insensitive, berated myself for being so screwed up about men, and told him it was over. Even though I was in a state of extreme despair, I was certain that I had discovered a snake in the grass, had gotten bitten, and that the only safe, not to mention smart, thing to do was to oust him. To do anything else would be to willingly invite a relationship with someone who was selfish and abusive.

Moving into My Insanity

But that wasn't how things panned out. I tried to break up with him, but it didn't work. Robert apologized and did his best to make it up to me. I let him back in, but this time I was sitting on an active volcano that would start spewing over any perceived slight. He'd switch over to another call for too long or spend time with his ex-boyfriend, I'd erupt, he'd try to make it up to me, and 'round and 'round we went.

Still, whenever I entered a thought-free zone, the good times could be so good. Dancing together was especially perfect—one time we had a spontaneous slow dance in my hallway to Barbra Streisand and Barry Gibb's "Guilty," and it was so sweet and fun and I felt extremely close to him. Though our physical relationship was pretty low key, Robert and I would spend time kissing and hugging in bed, and one time we lay there in my room and I felt a door open to some deeper part of myself I didn't know existed. For just a minute I thought it could be that, despite my fears, Robert and I might actually really be meant to be together.

Shortly after that he told me that he was going to end the "dating" and physical part of our relationship until he got clear about his feelings for his ex-boyfriend. Never mind that I was constantly trying to break up with him, or that now that I knew him and loved him I was no longer sexually attracted to him, or that I was so upset at him all the time that I often couldn't stand to be around him—I still felt completely rejected, sad and insanely furious.

I also became enraged at the way he lived his life and would be so upset at him and everything that was wrong with him and everything that he was doing wrong to me and every way that I wasn't getting what I deserved that, for the first time in my life, I couldn't sleep. And let me tell you, I need my sleep.

I finally decided one day months into this that I needed to break up with him for real this time. Consulting with a close girlfriend who saw things entirely from my perspective, she looked at me all red faced and teary eyed from feeling so ripped apart by the idea of ending my relationship with him altogether and said so softly while holding her hand over her heart, "Chris, you need to do this because you have to protect yourself."

And right there, I stopped and looked up in the middle of my sad little show.

Protect myself? Protect what exactly?

My breakup attempt failed again when he showed up with flowers and a beautiful book, and so we continued on, back on the merry-go-round of hell. But now I was unable to enjoy his company at all. No more sweet, slow dances in the hallway to '70s disco songs. The parts of me that hated him were squashing the parts of me that loved him, and I was unable to comprehend what I wanted—to invite him into that deepest part of me or to oust him from my life altogether.

Then one day he came to me while I was at work and told me he was losing his apartment and had nowhere to go. I stood there and looked into his face. My mind and body were quite still, and I heard the silent voice of knowledge very clearly tell me that the correct path was to invite him to move in. And, despite all the emotional chaos of our relationship, with a great sense of peace and clarity I did.

Losing My Mind and Having Nowhere to Run

Before Robert moved in I managed to get really excited. I love to be a host, and my only expectation is that people enjoy it. At least, that's what I thought.

As soon as he moved in I became a monster. I raged at him about dirty dishes, shoes left out in the hallway, my bed being unmade and his artwork left on the kitchen table. I smoldered in jealousy over any successes with his own projects, any rewards for his talents, positive beliefs he held about himself or any sexual attention he said he received.

The voices in my head tore him to pieces: he was emotionally immature, he was full of himself, he didn't know how to be intimate with someone he loved, he was withholding sex and love from me, he wasn't nearly as fabulous as he thought he was, he was only interested in trashy guys, he was a financial mess, he was using me, he was destroying my home life, and on and on.

I also secretly burned up with fury because he believed that I was a pathetic older sexual predator only helping him out so I could get him into bed. I was absolutely *sure* that he thought this, and I stewed over it for hours at a time.

But no matter how hard I tried to get him to conform or come up with a belief system about him that would ease my pain I couldn't *feel good* anymore. I hurt pretty much all the time.

Naturally, I blamed Robert for my insanity. And I was so blind with rage over the pain he was causing me that I could not acknowledge the numerous ways he showed his love and appreciation, such as by holding my hand as I woke up in the morning, greeting me at the door with a hug and a kiss, making beautiful pieces of art for me to give as gifts, and taking care of me whenever I got sick. One time he came to give me a very gentle kiss on the cheek good-bye while I was meditating, and I literally jumped off of my stool shouting at him for interrupting my peace. Needless to say it was a long time before he ever came up and gave me a kiss good-bye again under any circumstances.

As the months went by I lost my sanity altogether in regard to Robert. Though I didn't see it that way, I myself had become abusive. Do you know that scene in *Mommie Dearest* when

Joan Crawford is beating Christina with the Ajax over the imagined dirty bathroom floor? Well, that was pretty damn close to the reality that I had created in my own home, right down to patrolling the apartment for dirt in the blue bathrobe that Robert had given me for Christmas.

Then, out of nowhere, having never had a headache before in my life, I had a migraine so bad that I thought it was a stroke. Robert, of course, went to the hospital with me. In shock from the event—the doctors thought it was a stroke or an aneurysm—and from the inability of the doctors to correctly diagnosis my symptoms so that I believed I might be dying or permanently disabled, I lay on my stretcher with doctors swarming around me and pins and needles going in every which way and cracked like an egg. As Robert held my hand I heard myself say with total deathbed conviction, "I love you, Robert. I love you. I don't mean to say the things I say or yell at you like I do. I love you. I love you."

Back at home, recovering from the migraine and a botched spinal tap that left me bedridden for a week, in no time my anger returned. Only now every time I had a negative thought I had a piercing pain in my head as if someone were jamming an electrode into nerve endings in my brain. At that point I could either face my negativity or go on medication that would turn me into a zombie. I could descend further into unconsciousness and continue to see Robert and our relationship as I had and lose my health and my sanity, or I could find the willingness to let go of all of that "knowledge" about what he was doing to me and open myself up to looking at this situation consciously.

So, as usual, with my mental and physical health truly on the line, I was finally motivated to redirect my attention from Robert and onto myself. What I uncovered was the real story.

Opening Up My Wounds and Taking a Close Look

First, as excruciating as it was to stop blaming Robert for my pain, I began to search for the hidden stories behind my reactions. I began to think of my apartment as the evil cave Yoda sends Luke to in the *Empire Strikes Back* in order to discover that "evil" is in fact not about destroying Darth Vader, but about eradicating evil in himself. Similarly, I had to realize that my pain did not emanate from Robert, but rather from me. Living in the cave meant I had no choice but to face this because I had nowhere to run. And I was in so much pain that I could not possibly survive if I didn't heal it.

At first this approach made me *more* insane than I already was because my senses were still telling me that it was Robert's fault, but I could no longer temporarily find relief by blaming him or yelling at him or telling him to get out. I couldn't even get my morphine by going out and picking someone up! I was really fucked. But it seems I have always required a crisis in order to finally change.

I first began to get some sanity and correct my perceptions by writing down all of my unconscious beliefs and "knowledge" about Robert and our relationship, in addition to every belief I could think about when it came to sex, relationships, society, my appearance, my father, my upbringing, giving, you name it. And what I saw came as a true shock.

On the pages of my journal I saw evidence of a snake pit of poisonous and conflicting ideas that were controlling my perceptions: he thinks he can destroy my apartment; he thinks he can use me; he thinks I'm not hot or good looking; he thinks I'm an older sexual predator who is only helping him out for sex; he thinks I'm not good enough to be someone's boyfriend; he thinks I want him; and he thinks I'm as abusive as his ex-boyfriend.

Seemed right to me! But whose thoughts were these, his or mine? The fact was that I thought these things, suffered the results, and was projecting it onto Robert.

And so I began to see the backstory, which was that Robert was not the one hurting me: I was hurting myself in his presence with what I told myself unconsciously. It didn't matter how insane the basis of my "knowledge" was (like the idea that I could hear his thoughts), it was absolutely true to me because I believed it, and I believed it because I had created it.

But the truth was that it wasn't him I was critical of and who was making me crazy, it was me. I was so gullible to my own projections onto him that it still took me weeks after he left his new passport on the kitchen table for me to see that he had lied about his age and was in fact *two years older than me*, not five years younger, to finally stop believing that he thought I was an older sexual predator! That is the power of fear—truth is irrelevant to it; what matters is that you created it, and that's all it needs to be true to you.

Healing My Wounds

In the course of my life, it was my seemingly sane and healthy reasoning to "oust" anyone who "hurt me" like I thought Robert was hurting me. And I was certain that 99 percent of people would agree that this was indeed healthy.

But this idea that other people were the abusers and that it was necessary to avoid them had not changed the repetitive "abusive" relationships I had in the form of people who upset me, let me down and didn't give me what I wanted. In fact, I simply kept creating the same relationships over and over—evolving, as Gary Zukav calls it in *The Seat of the Soul*, horizontally rather than vertically so that the externals changed, but the fundamental issues within me repeated themselves over and over like a broken record.

And Robert was many of these repetitive relationships wrapped up in one: he was my father messing up my house and making me feel powerless; he was every gay guy who had "rejected" me; he was everyone I had ever helped who had "used me"; and ultimately he was everyone else in the world who had decided that I would never get my due because I was not good enough.

He was also everything I hated about myself. All those criticisms I had of him personally were all projections of my own inner voices, which were constantly trying to tell me how pathetic I really was underneath my fabulous costume. This was why I couldn't accept him for who he was—I didn't accept myself.

Usually with even one of these issues uncovered I'd break up with the guy and tell him I never wanted to see him again because *he* was too unstable. This time around I did the opposite: I invited the experience in order to finally evolve vertically by learning what I was supposed to learn—that I was the one who was hurting myself, and that I had a choice to stop if I wanted to.

Looking at my painful relationship with him this way, for the first time I began to understand that the reason I couldn't see Robert for Robert anymore nor understand our relationship with any clarity was because I was on an endless search to ambush Robert and prove that he was doing these things to me. This is the awesome power of perception at work: it only allows in what it already believes to be true.

Bringing this hidden snake pit into the light was the first step in being able to understand my reactions to Robert clearly, because suddenly I had the eyes to see how I was interpreting events according to these unconscious ideas. In other words, the veil began to lift, and I began to see a lot of powerful truths about what was really going on.

Realizing the Difference Between Love and Fear

The truth was that I wasn't on the verge of tears over Robert nor desperate for Robert to "choose" me over his ex-boyfriend because I was in love with him or because I was tuned in to some innate knowledge that we were supposed to be together. The fact is that I was terrified he was pulling his love and acceptance away like I feared all men would eventually do. Similarly, I wasn't jealous over his attraction to other men because of love, but rather because in those moments I withdrew love and acceptance of myself because I thought I was not meeting *his* image of perfection when in fact it was my own that I didn't match up to.

There were many other beliefs that I disguised as love but that had nothing whatsoever to do with love . . . at least not love for him. I had an unconscious belief that Robert was supposed to make me happy and give me unconditional love and acceptance, even though I didn't extend it to him; that his success at anything meant failure for me; that he was the only good guy out there for me, and if I didn't get him I'd never get anyone; and that any time he "messed up" my apartment in any way he was trying to destroy me like I believed my father had.

And though it is true that I was very giving to Robert—something I reminded him about relentlessly—I had an unconscious belief that if I gave anything, especially to a love interest, I was supposed to get something back, and if I didn't, he was "using me." I was also blaming him for my decision to help him out. Underlying all of this was a firm belief in scarcity; I believed that Robert was taking away from my incredibly finite resources, not just money, time and space, but love.

Finally I realized what my good girlfriend had meant when she said I needed to protect myself. It wasn't me I needed to protect, it was all these wounds I had which he had touched unwittingly. Not realizing this, I was taking the usual route of trying to correct something in myself by trying to correct Robert and masking it as love. But correcting him in order to correct something in myself would never work and the whole idea was totally insane.

The hardest fact to realize about our relationship was that I was nowhere near ready to be in a conscious, loving relationship with sex. Neither was he. We couldn't have been further from it, but I was blaming him for not being able to do what I myself couldn't do. I couldn't see this and accept him and accept myself because I was wrapping all my garbage, all my pain and all my fears in the auspices of "love"—with the notion that if only he would love me properly my pain would go away. I did love him deeply, but I had confused all my other garbage with love, too, to the point that I couldn't even feel my actual love anymore. What I needed to do was give up all that horrible pain disguising itself as romantic "love," which was hiding me from the truth, and use this relationship in order to heal myself and thereby heal our relationship.

Robert was the perfect teacher, and my apartment was the perfect classroom for me to finally take this lesson. That was the truth of our relationship, and that was what I recognized when

I met him. Recognizing the true meaning of our relationship meant I recognized that it was indeed a perfect relationship because it was tailor-made for my healing.

How I'd Hidden My Wounds from Myself

One of the reasons these wounds were unknown to me was because I didn't want anyone, including myself, to know about them. It was as if my positive image of myself and my anger were a lion at the gate that distracted attention from the wounded, bleeding me behind the bars—I only wanted the world to see the lion at the gate, and I wanted to believe I was him, too. I realized as well that, when I was in high school, instead of a lion there had been a beggar holding out his cup for charity.

I thought I'd made it when the lion replaced the beggar. That was the entire concept behind creating a "new me" every few years that projected an image of myself that I was in no pain and, in fact, had it all. This was my idea of self-love, and no doubt, as my supernaturally brilliant therapist, Christine Ranck, points out, the only way I knew to survive. And it was a necessary step. We always have to work with what we know at any given time, and my only real sense of self-love was through an illusory grasp at external acceptance. But little did I know all I'd done was alter the illusion so that I couldn't see I was still a deeply hurt person.

And this is an incredibly common defense mechanism. I know so many gay men who are perfect "lions"—they look amazing, they never crack in public, and the press release on themselves is that they aren't hurt and they don't have any emotional problems or weaknesses. Often they are not consciously aware that they are in any pain at all. For all they know they really are telling the truth because they have both walled themselves off from it and also become so numb to the throbbing undercurrent of hurt in their lives that they don't even know it's there anymore. When I hear their lion's roar of denial over any suggestion that there may be more to what they're feeling than they acknowledge—one buddy of mine actually told me that he doesn't have any emotional struggles at all—I hear myself, and I remember exactly what that was like.

Healing My Relationship by Healing Myself

The only way to begin to change the toxic dynamic between me and Robert was to drop my lion act and change my intent in our relationship. Up until this point my unconscious intent was to enforce my old "reality" of external hurt and external acceptance by blaming Robert for how I felt. My new intent was to heal myself and thereby my relationship with Robert, whatever the outcome might be and at risk of whatever I thought I might "lose."

To heal these wounds I had to correct the misperceptions that caused them. My new and clear line of vision revealed the essential truth behind my toxic relationship with Robert, which was that I would only stop attacking him when I stopped attacking myself.

Waking up from the dream that it's other people who hurt me was one of the most difficult struggles of my entire life. Facing how deep my wounds really were has also been brutal because I thought those wounds meant I was weak. I thought they were true. I thought they were me. Now I know they are not me, and they have nothing whatsoever to do with love. In fact, they are the opposite of love because it is in not loving yourself that you wound yourself.

What has occurred—and is still occurring every day—after all of this work is nothing less than a miracle: as I began to heal myself with these truths I began to heal my relationship with Robert. From a place of hysteria, insanity and contradiction, I slowly found myself in a zone of calm, sanity and wisdom.

Step by step, day by day I felt my love begin to come out again, and I was able to enjoy his company once more. As I criticized myself less I criticized him less and felt love again. When we went out together to a New Year's Eve party and we finally danced together again—this time to the Bee Gees "Stayin' Alive"—I knew we were healing. And when I found myself stopping at the kitchen table to gaze at his artwork because I was so astounded by his talent and so grateful that he was close to me, I knew I was feeling my love again and that we could manage to be close after all.

And this isn't easy, because as a wounded lion, you cannot have a close relationship. Closeness gets you close to your wounds, which, as a lion, you are not even willing to accept are there. My good friend's ex-boyfriend, like a lot of lions I know, doesn't have a single actual intimate relationship in his life: his relationships of all kinds are very fragile and very temporary because the second someone gets close to a wound—usually for him it's by not giving him enough attention—he cuts them out of his life right away and moves on to the next superficial relationship. He's got his pride, but he's got no love and no intimacy.

Making the Distinction Between Love and Pain, and Discovering the Source of Love

In the process of all this excavating, I came to, and continue to come to, profound realizations about the nature and source of my pain and dysfunction in my relationships. I understand now that it's not love that hurts, it's pain and fear. They've been confused to such a point that we are all trained to believe that love is pain, which is, if you listen closely, the message behind practically every pop song you've ever heard: loving you hurts me, not having you hurts me, losing you hurts me, if only I had you I could stop hurting. The word in the music is always "love," but what they are referring to is in fact *pain*. This insane notion is why most of the guys I know think they've really fallen in love when the thought of the guy they're into causes them pain. I've been there, too. The prevailing idea that we are all raised with is that a lot of pain equals being in love.

But this is not the case. Pain is pain and it hurts. Fear is fear and it hurts because it causes pain. Love is love and it feels wonderful. Making the distinction between love and pain is the first step to sanity. Another is to realize not just the source of pain, but the source of love. It is not, as pop songs and Hollywood films would have you believe, that it is the other person's love you feel or the other person who withholds love from you—it is your own love that you either allow yourself to feel or not.

For me realizing this has meant that I am no longer in search of someone to love me properly, but rather on the inner search to release and feel my own love without conditions. Relationships are no longer strained with the expectation that the other person love me, but are rather practices for me to share in the abundance of my own love, which is the only love I could ever feel in the first place, which is, in fact, the one "macro" love that I and you and everyone individually are "micros" of.

Healing myself by realizing that it was my own painful thoughts that I heard and believed—not Robert's—and my own love that I either gave myself or withheld, helped me begin to understand these truths through direct experience. I decided to *never* deny myself love, happiness and sanity over anything again. After all, nothing I did had anything to do with Robert but rather with my own issues. Everything Robert did had to do with his issues. Neither was a good excuse to withhold love from myself.

Understanding this meant there was nothing to take personally and no reason to not love and give selflessly out of my own simple desire to be happy and share my own abundant resources of love. With this, I realized I could never be "used" by anyone because my love cannot ever be diminished or used up. Giving is my choice, and my happiness.

Just as this ended the "romantic" ideals of my relationship with Robert, this realization might seriously alter the dynamic of your existing "romantic" relationships. My friend David was always certain that whomever he was dating was withholding love from him, and that the pain he felt over this was equated with the pain of being "in love." After all, love hurts. But in his last such relationship he began to realize that it was his own love that he withheld from or gave to himself based on whether the guy called or didn't call, wanted to sleep with him or didn't want to sleep with him, and so on, which is what he had experienced with every guy he ever dated, over and over and over. Once he stepped into sanity he realized that he wasn't "in love" with the guy, and in fact he didn't love him at all. Though that ended their dating relationship—and the painful "in love" pattern he'd been in his whole life that caused him to suffer so much—it was also what allowed him to actually love the guy. In learning how to allow his own love to flow abundantly, he was able to share it even though they were no longer dating.

Watching All of My Relationships Heal

As I worked to heal my wounds and changed my practice with people from one focused on getting love from them to one of learning and of sharing my love, the black cloud over my relationships with everyone in the world from strangers and old enemies to close friends and homeless people began to transform. I began and am continuing to evolve vertically. I know this because my relationships have changed. I have witnessed my relationships with men, both straight and gay, transform into meaningful, authentic expressions of inspiration, consciousness, honesty and closeness. And this is really a first for me since I first became poisoned about men twenty-five years ago.

The key to evolving vertically has been in my willingness to switch from *taking* from people to *giving*. The more healed the less I was in need and the less I needed to take my acceptance or happiness or my due from Robert or anyone else. I was able to switch more and more to giving, and therein find my sanity and my happiness. After all, when you are in a state of loss, you need to take. In a state of abundance, the imperative is to give. It's that simple.

A couple of years later I vertically ascended to my next level of healing in a relationship I developed with my friend Sagi. As Sagi woke up from a deep state of unconsciousness, he suffered tremendously as he stripped away his cover-ups and felt the excruciating pain he'd been in since he was a child. He was like a burn victim in a trauma unit going off the morphine, and as a result he had nothing to give back, including love or attention, and yet he required almost constant nurturing. But I had enough love to give, and I didn't expect anything in return.

But as he healed his most horrific, lifelong wounds and began to let go of his defenses, our relationship blossomed into a fantastically reciprocal practice for both of us to love each other selflessly and help each other wake up. And as he continued to heal more and more he became very giving to me, to the point that the first thing out of his mouth is usually an offer of some kind. What I learned from this beautiful and perfect relationship with him is that in having enough love to share, I naturally invite people who want to share theirs with me. This is the nature of a perfect relationship, and the gift that was waiting behind the door of selfless service to another person. I'm not trying to say that I'm a saint, but rather that we are all saints in disguise, and each of us has the capacity to give in extreme abundance, and in doing so, receive even more.

This next stage was exactly what I needed in order to get on the path to having a healthy wonderful relationship with a man with whom I am also having sex *because it is all the same*—every beautiful relationship that works has the same ingredients: self-love, self-acceptance, selfless giving, and an absence of fear. If you get it right in one relationship (as I get it right with Sagi) you can get it right in every relationship.

This turning of the page in the way I experience myself has allowed me to become vulnerable again in a healthy, sane, real and intimate way, and, in doing so, truly invulnerable for I realize that I have everything essential and also that I have nothing to lose because *I will not hurt myself.* Sagi and I put this into practice endlessly because whenever either one of us feels hurt by the other, we put the attention on ourselves, find the source, heal it and then move on. And it's work. But as a result, I now know what closeness with a man is actually like, and it is such a beautiful thing.

Now I am beginning to perceive myself, and everyone and

everything in the world through love, which is the very basis for sanity and happiness.

Heal Your Wounds

I am not going to pretend that going though this journey has not been a truly harrowing and painful venture, or that it doesn't continue to be difficult. Quite frankly, it often feels like surgery without anesthesia. But you have to realize that your anesthesia and avoidances are a part of the problem because you have to *feel* what is wrong in order to recognize it. You cannot feel your pain when you have anesthetized it with phony relationships, a closet full of Dolce & Gabbana, a "masculine" or "feminine" image, drugs (prescription or otherwise), tricks, or with an Internet ad indicating how beautiful, masculine, distant, invulnerable, romantic, un-gay or oversexed you are.

As a matter of fact, to heal begins with pain, for the pain tells you there is something to heal. The analogy Don Miguel Ruiz makes in *The Mastery of Love* is to wounds on your skin: if your skin is healthy, a touch feels good. If it is wounded, a touch feels bad and you recoil. People touch us all the time—not just by speaking to us but by their sheer existence. But it's not their fault whether you hurt or feel good, because it's always about you.

When you feel the pain from wounds, your natural reaction is a desire to not feel it. At that point, you have two choices: to take the route into deeper unconsciousness by covering up or avoiding the pain, or to go through it and feel it in order to heal by bringing the causes into conscious awareness. Most of the time when it's a physical wound we choose to heal it, but for some reason when it's an emotional wound we want to cover it up. But covering up emotional wounds is no more sane than covering up a broken leg and then blaming someone else when they touch it.

If you choose to cure yourself, and thereby heal your love and relationships, you must do the deep excavating of your old fears, hopes and belief systems that make the pain happen. *You have to give up the "knowledge" that anyone ever hurt you emotionally and find out what you are telling yourself that is causing your pain.* You also have to give up the idea that your love is "out there" in someone else; it is, in fact, sitting right inside you waiting to be felt. The following are the steps to take to heal yourself, the love that you feel and the relationships that you have.

Step One: Decide to Heal

Healing begins with a decision. It requires a desire to rid yourself of the pain forever, a true desire to heal your relationships, discover intimacy and release your love, and a willingness to let go of every way in which you have perceived yourself and the world up until now. This is the moment you choose to wake up during a crisis instead of fall into a deeper sleep. Like my turning point with depression, it is the moment that you rebel. As Eckhart Tolle put it in *The Power of Now*, when threatened, unconscious people fall into deeper unconsciousness, while conscious people use it as a means to becoming more conscious. Being conscious, you will respond to threats as a chance to heal, which means you take the first step toward evolving vertically into new dimensions rather than evolving horizontally and repeating the same old cycles.

This decision to heal requires a new and conscious intent. Your old, unconscious intent was to cover up and avoid your wounds and to have total faith that it was other people who hurt you and other people who held your happiness and love in their hands. Your new intent is to consider that the only way to heal your pain is to reconsider this idea.

Step Two: Recognize Your Pain as Your Pain

Having decided to heal, you must now begin to recognize your pain as *your pain*. This includes not interpreting "wounds" as metaphorical—they are as real as the pain that you feel. No matter how justified you feel about being negative, you realize that your negativity, your pain, is yours and that you are the one suffering. After all, where does your pain take place? Where do you feel your negativity? Whose horrible thoughts do you hear? It's all you.

This sounds easy, but it's actually quite difficult. We automatically react by focusing on an external who or what that "caused" us pain because that is what we want to believe. In fact it's a matter of who or what has *revealed* our pain, which is ours and nobody else's, to us.

Think of it this way: if someone says something to offend you that is blatantly untrue, you will not be hurt. You will just think that person is crazy, and it clearly has nothing to do with you. But if someone calls you a "faggot" and you are hurt, it is because part of you believes you are what the word "faggot" implies to you. It is your pain that is called up and exposed, and they have touched it with their words, and this is what you must begin to recognize.

Step Three: Look for How You Cover Up or Avoid Your Pain

This next step is crucial in the deconstruction of your illusions of pain and hurt because at this stage you are going to begin to see your negative reactions for what they truly are. You will unmask violent emotions, manipulative tactics and old habits to reveal their true nature, which is your pain with a mask. The point is that unless you strip away the outer layers of your defense mechanisms you will not be able to hear and feel what is really going on underneath. But as you do you will be able to tune in to the stories you are telling yourself that color what you see, create the emotional reactions you don't understand nor consciously want, and which result in very dissatisfying relationships.

This is a big project. You have been covering up your pain for years and reacting habitually whenever your wounds have been touched. You have also created avoidance mechanisms so that you don't put yourself at risk of anyone touching them. The result has been lots of drama, breakups, stress, fear, addictions, tears, loneliness, sadness, worry, anxiety, avoidances, listlessness, confusion, cocooning, depression, fights, hysteria, insanity, retributions, retaliations . . . need I go on? The point is that to cure them you have to start seeing the cover-ups and avoidances as such.

It also means that whereas you once thought of your panic attacks or depression solely as a chemical problem and your best hope was for a pill that could numb you enough that you would have a semblance of a life again, you begin to see them as symptoms of your wounds that can be healed. This is a weighty issue to many people, but if you have any doubts at all that thoughts create your emotions, consider that all thoughts have emotional results—when I thought I wasn't good enough, I was depressed. When I stopped thinking that, I stopped being depressed. Or, for instance, I have two friends who have suffered greatly from panic attacks. One has not yet been able to face his demons, and he can't function without the antidepressants that quell the panic. The other also had hideous panic attacks but chose to face the cause and found the source in an unconscious terror of being abandoned. Healing that fear, he now has no more panic attacks because he no longer perceives anything to be panicked over. Trust me, you've got the power to heal yourself, too.

You'll have to figure out what cover-ups and avoidance mechanisms you've got. And the answer is not in the action itself, but rather the revelation is in discovering the intent to cover and avoid your wounds that might lie behind the action.

Here are some usual suspects to look out for: anger; staying busy; never being alone; always being alone; trying to change others; being judgmental, sanctimonious and critical; grudges; repetitive breakups; achievement; taking things personally; morphine in the form of approval; sex sites that offer a twenty-four-hour-a-day morphine drip; false humility; feeling sorry for yourself; self-imposed limits; narcissism; anonymous sex; anonymous relationships; the need to be right; drugs and alcohol; masking wounds as love so that rejection in the form of jealousy, obsession and possessiveness get confused with love; your image; passive aggressiveness, manipulations and defensive living; and finally societal expectations of all sorts because it's easier to live out a false external expectation of a relationship than to feel anything real.

Step Four: Refrain from Reacting, Feel Your Pain and Learn What Is Causing It

After you have begun to see your avoidances and cover-ups for what they are, you must then begin to refrain from acting on them. This does not mean you will not continue to feel the impulses—oh, if only. You will continue to feel them until the wounds are healed. But this time around, you do so consciously because you know them for what they are. So it's not just that you learn to think clearly, you learn to *feel* clearly because you can finally properly identify emotions for what they actually are, not what they might first seem to be.

For instance, once you recognize anger as pain with a mask and the desperate need to pick up a trick as the pressing of your morphine button, you start seeing the symptoms of *your pain* whenever anger or the desperate need for a pickup arises. With your new intent to heal in mind, you choose then to refrain from acting on your old cover-up reactions.

Refraining is one of the most difficult parts of the healing process because this is willingly giving up the anesthesia and the avoidances. No doubt there is withdrawal—my friend who healed his panic attacks had to actually go through the panic instead of going out and meeting a guy in order to find out what was behind it and then heal it. But refraining is the only way you can feel your pain and find out what stories, beliefs and fears have caused it. Feeling pain also becomes a major motivation to heal it.

The difficulty of refraining is directly proportional to the power that is released from it. By refraining you begin to see that you are *not* your reactions: *you* are not anger, insatiable horniness, desperation, panic, depression or any other number of feelings you were being victimized by. In a miraculous feat of transformation, you begin to see that you experience these things, but *are* none of them because you watch them come, then you watch them go, and you are still there.

I only suggest that you do your best on this. Do not judge yourself if you indulge an unconscious reaction or are overcome by an unconscious reaction. I am not suggesting that, as my friend Valerie says, you "spiritualize away your feelings" by telling yourself that because you are working to be conscious you should not have certain feelings. I only mean that you set your intent to do your best to refrain and learn from unconscious reactions rather than being victimized by them, that's all. Just do your best and then let go. During the whole process treat yourself as gently and lovingly as you would a baby learning how to walk, and you'll really be on your way.

From this new perspective you begin to see the unconscious negative patterns of your life such as addiction, depression or loneliness that have been in control of you, and then release them.

To successfully get to a place where refraining from your habitual reactions is a habit in and of itself, you must not only practice it a lot—for practice makes perfect—but you must also follow the learning curve. In other words, you see that someone says or does something to cause a habitual pain covering-up reaction and the first thing you feel is the *heat* of that reaction—whether it's anger, horniness, manipulation, cocooning, whatever—and you realize that you have to first focus on letting that heat cool down.

Often this means sitting in your room by yourself smoldering over some injustice or melting in depression but keeping it to yourself until the passion of the reaction has faded. It may be even harder than you expected when you observe that part of you protects the pain because you made it and it is precious to you. Any way you slice it you give yourself the time, and you recognize that this is part of the process. You find the will to do it because you don't see the mask anymore, you see your pain.

Then, once your reaction has cooled down, you begin to ask yourself the tough questions. Why am I angry at my boss for not giving me my Christmas bonus? Why am I dying to get on the Internet and pick someone up? Why do I want a snort of crystal or a hit of X so badly? Why do I want to get depressed? Why am I so nauseated by that group of gay men that I can't stand to be around them? Why did I want to yell at my boyfriend? Why am I so threatened by my brother's ideas about religion? Why do I feel it is necessary to withhold from my boyfriend how much I love him? Why am I dishing so much guilt out on my closest friend? Why, why, why?

Once you start to answer those questions, you get to the feeling-your-pain part because you have refrained from covering it up. And you find that one moment you were the lion (or even the beggar) and now you are the wounded person behind the facade you've been hiding from others and yourself. Now you come to the pain you have been covering up.

My roommate Dean has suffered from terrible anxiety attacks his whole life but has recently begun to observe and refrain from giving into them, which is an incredibly brave thing to do. In doing so he's found the source of his anxiety in the form of terrible fear that he's going to appear incompetent, and which can be exposed with as tiny a thing as spilling a glass of water. By observing his reaction he has discovered a part of himself that believes he doesn't know what he's doing. In becoming aware of this belief and releasing it, he is slowly healing the anxiety.

In dealing with your own reactions, even though you're probably still desperately wanting to hate someone for what they think about you, you have to sit there and change the grammar in your thoughts from, "He thinks he can just use me on the side while he gives all of his attention to his boyfriend," to "*I think* he can just use me on the side while he gives all of his attention to his boyfriend."

The way to end this type of painful thinking is to find out what fears you are harboring that form thoughts such as these that we then project onto others. You have to learn what hopes and expectations you are projecting onto relationships and what story lines are playing themselves out again and again in your life, for these illusions and misperceptions are the sources of your pain.

First you look for specific unconscious beliefs about the situation that has called up the pain. They're there, but we aren't conscious of them, so it requires digging.

To become conscious of my unconscious beliefs I generally work first with leading questions for myself. Say I met a cute guy and he acted so interested, asked me out, then blew me off, and I was hurt. I might begin by asking myself, "By blowing me off it means . . ." and filling in that blank. Say that answer is, "He doesn't think I'm attractive enough to bother." Then I would continue by saying, "If he doesn't think I'm attractive, then I'm not attractive," which leads to, "I'm afraid I'm not attractive." Further I would say, "And if I'm not attractive then I'm who I was in middle school—I'm not lovable, and I will be all alone and left out." Eventually by following the trail I wind up at some place inside of me that says, "If I'm not attractive and lovable to others, then I won't love myself."

And bam, I've come to the real reason I'm upset. It's not

because he might have been "the one" (which my friend Sagi brilliantly termed "the ultimate in scarcity") or because I'm constantly being blown off by men. It is my own hurt I'm causing myself and that is being exposed through someone else's actions. And believe me, the guy didn't call for his own damn reasons that have nothing to do with me.

You are the only one who can follow the bread-crumb trail of your story lines, but now you know how to do it. Once you do follow that trail deep enough, you discover deeper and more general damaging beliefs. You may believe that because you have HIV you *are* HIV, and so you are unlovable; that black men are superior to white men and because you are white you are inferior; that white men are superior to black men and because you are black you are inferior; that you're too old and messed up for anyone to love; that you will only love yourself if you have a thirty-two-inch waist; that you cannot be happy unless you have a boyfriend; or that no one would want to know you out of drag.

We tell ourselves these things, we believe them, events "prove" them to be true, then we are hurt, and then we bring that hurt into every single relationship in the world, simultaneously trying to prove them and disprove them while other people get shaken around like rag dolls by all of our unconscious garbage. Meanwhile we perpetrate a huge lie on others that all of our jealousy and possessiveness have to do with them because we love them, when it has nothing at all to do with loving others, but everything to do with the fact that you believe these horrible things, and so you do not love yourself.

In following the bread-crumb trail, you then find it gets even deeper than that. Each expression of fear and pain eventually winds up at a foundational fear, idea, expectation and story line.

What is problematic in negotiating your way through this maze is that our belief systems are set up in such a way that they do not appear to be beliefs at all—they are taken to be reality. In fact they are simply *unquestioned assumptions.* Therefore they are difficult to even locate to question. This is especially true because we project them onto the world by saying, "People hate gay men," or "Nobody thinks overweight people are attractive." Isn't this the case? You'd be crazy to not see it! But behind that is a choice, too, as Don Miguel Ruiz says in *The Four Agreements,* to *agree* with these sentiments. In other words, you're the one who has chosen to believe it, and that is what makes it real to you.

In asking yourself what is the truth behind your pain, look for beliefs in scarcity of both physical resources and intangible resources such as love and happiness; a concept of "the one" in the form of one person "out there" who is holding your love and happiness, and if you don't find him you will never have either; a desire to "own" people you find beautiful or perfect; fears that create insatiable appetites for what we already have, such as fears of rejection, of being alone, of being used, not getting what you deserve and of having your happiness taken away; expectations about how you or others should be; decisions not to love yourself under certain conditions; unwillingness to accept others for who they are; beliefs that you are not perfect because you are gay, or white, Chinese, or an insurance salesman; decisions to put limits on whom you will love; conflicting ideas about yourself such as that you are incredibly smart and unbelievably stupid; and the idea that you have no control over your own life.

These are just a few suggestions, and as usual you will have to discover your own snake pit. By bringing these unconscious beliefs into conscious awareness, you will realize that you have been poisoned by their bites. You will also discover that you thought *you* were that poison. In shining your light there, you will rid yourself of that snake pit and begin to heal from its poisonous effects on your system, on your relationships and on your very being.

You'll also discover that you have not been the victim of someone else's abuse but the victim of your own unconscious abuse. You created each relationship. You created the feelings. Everything was there that you needed to learn to move on. It was you all along.

Step Five: Correct Your Vision

Now that you realize that it was problems in how you perceived yourself and your relationships all along, not other people and their problems, how do you begin to see things accurately? The great thing is that all you have to do is not have incorrect vision in order to have correct vision. Once you begin to know yourself, which is the still observer of all of this, you will be able to know others and to decide consciously what kind of relationship you want with anyone you meet. You didn't know people for who they were before, and you always got a lot of unhappy surprises when the facade collapsed and their snakes began to bite you and your snakes fought back. This is how relationships with guys who seemed "so nice" at first and whom you felt such incredible passion for could collapse into nothingness, or even horror.

Now you can see people for who they are because you know who you are, which means you'd only choose to have an intimate relationship with someone you felt was ready for one.

Before, you saw a body, projected your unconscious movie and cast them in a role they don't even know they're playing. Now you perceive a soul and feel vibrations of attraction all over your being. It's a big difference, and the ability to do this comes from self-knowledge.

Getting there does often mean inviting painful relationships and evolving in them. That's because you always have to start where you are right now. This is what I did with Robert, and it's how I grew. Without Robert I would still be extremely angry and isolated when it came to men. I would also not have been in the place to write this book. If you're a lion like me it's scary because you're used to avoiding these situations. If you're a beggar you're used to thinking you have nothing and are lucky even to get abused. Either way evolving is like standing in the middle of a fire long enough to realize that there is no fire.

Of course many people will disagree with your path to correct your vision because they will interpret it from their own unconscious viewpoint. This is yet another challenge to your journey toward wakefulness, but their words and opinions will only resonate in you to the degree that you still agree with them. Use their challenges to your journey ("I'm sorry, if you stay with that guy you are a chump!" "You wouldn't be so obsessed with him if you weren't really in love!") as a means to expose your old programming running in your mind and an opportunity to start living your life like you want to, not like the cult tells you to.

The next step, once you have really begun to see the truth and to heal, is to create other healing relationships, but this time start off consciously, authentically and selflessly with healing as your intent. Then, much to your surprise, one day you're going to look up and realize that you've created a heavenly relationship and you didn't even realize it! You didn't recognize it because it took place outside of the cult, and you had no words or categories to understand it.

It will still be work—hidden snakes will still reveal themselves to you and your conscious partners. You spend a beautiful weekend at the beach together having so much fearless fun, then one of you brings back the wrong Popsicle for the other, and ten minutes later you aren't speaking and you wonder, oh my God, am I going to lose this one, too? But this time you both practice consciousness with each other so it no longer turns into a horror show. Together you can practice helping and loving each other selflessly. In this relationship one of you will be able to expose yourself by saying, "I got upset that you brought the wrong Popsicle because you didn't apologize, which calls up my fear that underneath it all you're just like every other asshole who hurt me." The other can look inside and say, "I didn't apologize because I have a fear that I'm dumb and can't do anything right, and I think if I apologize for being wrong that I'm admitting that I'm an idiot."

Then you can both apologize for taking it personally and go back to loving each other, though this time you feel even closer because you have demonstrated to each other that the other person is more important to you than being right. Believe it or not, this is a typical conversation I have with Sagi and now even Robert. The truth always diffuses negativity because the truth is always harmless.

The point is that neither of you take anything personally, both of you are thinking more about the other than yourself, both of you want to show who you really are, and both of you prioritize your relationship and your love for the other high enough that you are willing to expose your weaknesses. Imagine that—someone in your life who is willing to love you and accept you even though you may in an unconscious moment be perceiving their love as an attack. And you've invited a person in who can give that to you because that's where you are, too.

To have a conscious relationship like this, it is mandatory that you give up your addiction to expectations in the form of "categories." For instance, programming that tells you that you should only have a beautiful relationship with a "romantic" partner is profoundly dangerous. That's because "romantic" essentially means that you not only limit your love to "the one" or the closest facsimile you can find, but also that you expect that person to be something that he isn't, which is your idea of romantic perfection, and that he does something that he can't, which is make you happy. And when he isn't and he doesn't because he can't, the relationship will go dark or fizzle out and he becomes, as Sagi calls it, just another "one of them."

"Romantic" is a great word to describe dancing to Sade on your rooftop underneath a starry sky, but other than that the word is a snake is disguise. After all, every romantic fantasy starts off, and ends, with loneliness. What the hell is romantic about that? You don't need it. Just remember this: romance didn't make the cosmos, love did.

For those who fear the end of romance, enlightenment doesn't mean you don't have special relationships anymore. Though it is the end of "the one" person "out there" holding your happiness and the beginning of having a hard time explaining your relationships to people because they no longer fit into the usual categories, what it really means to you is that *every* relationship becomes special whether you have a mate or not. Beauty and meaning enter into every transaction, whether social, sexual, professional, personal, temporary, immediate, distant, what have you, because through every person God is speaking to you, telling you exactly what you need to hear by showing you exactly what you need to learn. You only need to tune out of all the "categories" in order to tune in to this voice.

The realization that God is in every person you see is the ultimate symptom of healing. You only arrive there when you make your own connection with your true nature: the very fact that you see God in everyone is a mirror of the fact that you feel you are a part of God as well. Your knowledge of anyone is directly proportional to how well you know yourself. In this state your vision becomes corrected. With correct vision you recognize that you have an infinite amount of love in you already so why in the world do you need to go *get it* from anyone else? The imperative in the case of infinite abundance is to share, so you can just take buckets of love and pour it over anyone's head because you've got nothing to lose.

Suddenly your relationships start to become magical. Before, people resonated on the vibe you gave out, which was one of unconscious manipulation, and indeed you invited in people who were "using" you just as you "used" them, which only proved your case that you were being used and that people couldn't be trusted.

Now relationships of that sort transform. The love for and acceptance of yourself is something you can freely give to others, so now not only do you find that you simply can't be used, you also find yourself in relationships in which both partners are giving. You begin to attract people on the same wavelength, so you now find yourself receiving as much abundance as you share.

After all this practice of seeing that love is not pain nor any of its disguises, you begin to experience what love actually is.

Though describing it is like describing an ocean because you have to see it and jump in in order to know it at all, from my own experiences I can describe it as the opposite of fear. It makes you feel that nothing is impossible and that life and the people in it are delicious, and there need not be any pain or loneliness at the beginning or the end of that rainbow. You realize there is no bad ending because you don't create one anymore. When you find yourself taking sheer joy in the love coming out of you rather than highs and lows based on the love you think is being given to you or being withheld, you'll know you've evolved vertically and realized real love.

When you boil it all down, it is *exactly* as RuPaul says: "If you don't love yourself, how in the hell are you going to love anybody else?" I used to think that was gobbledygook. Now I see the truth of it. Jesus put it this way: "Love thy neighbor as thyself." He didn't just mean it as a commandment, he meant it as a statement of fact—you can only love people exactly according to how much love you have for yourself.

In correcting your vision by bringing all of your unconscious beliefs and fears into the light, you also discover you had lots of unconscious and conflicting intents. Like my friend David who was sure his whole life that he really wanted intimate relationships but then realized that he only picked people who dealt exclusively on the surface. Or like me, though I thought all I wanted was easy sex, underneath it all was a hope I'd meet Mr. Right who would make me feel perfect.

You get the exact result conflicted intents result in, which is conflict. As you end the conflict by creating whole and conscious intents you find out what it is you really want in any relationship. You can extend yourself fearlessly because instead of acting on the illusion of scarcity, you now give in to the realization of abundance. And I don't mean abundance of material goods or hot men—I mean, as my close friend Joaquin defines it, as "an abundance of anything you need to share your light."

When you move on you also no longer spend time focusing on what is wrong with everyone else—if your boyfriend regularly hangs up the phone on you in fits of anger, you don't *have* to make him change. You don't tell yourself that his action means you aren't significant because you are conscious of your inherent and indestructible significance. You can just ask yourself, can I have a conscious relationship with someone with that much unresolved selfishness and anger? Maybe, maybe not. But staying with him or changing the relationship won't be about proving you matter because you *know* you matter regardless of how he acts. And if he's upsetting you, then you can heal what he's calling up, see him for who he is, not for what you are afraid he means about you, and then make a conscious decision about whether this is the type of relationship you want. There are plenty of amazing relationships out there for you to have, so you don't ever have to worry about moving from there into nothing if you decide to make a change.

Everyone likes to talk about how much the world needs love, but few are willing to do the work to release their own because it's tough and it's painful. When you see how hard it is, you begin to see why the world is so absent of love. Look around and ask yourself if the prevailing ideas of love and relationships are working. If you see hell on Earth, then you can also find your will to change there because just as hell and pain travel, so does heaven and love: you realize yours, you share it, and it spreads. Trust me, you will see it spread and feel so good.

It takes true heroes to wage the only true war there is, which is the one inside of ourselves. If you do this work you're going to go through a lot, no doubt. Your love has been clogged up for a very long time because you taught yourself that love hurts. Now you see that it wasn't love that hurt, it was fear. People don't wear their hearts on their sleeves, they wear their pain, which they cause themselves and then blame others. By healing the parts of you that need to heal, you're going to rediscover love for what it really is, for love, happiness and acceptance are like petals off the same bloom. If you have one, you have them all. And one day your heart is going to crack open like an egg and all that love that was clogged up is going to come pouring out. And then you're going to know what real happiness is all about.

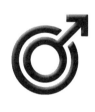

6

Homophobia: The True Path to Liberation Is Internal

As we're liberated from our own fear, our presence automatically liberates others.

—Marianne Williamson

By this point you already know my story and everything essential to conscious living. As you can see, each part is integrated—no subject is separate from another, nor is any truth for one any different from a truth for another. It is all the same.

I have also already indicated that the way to freedom is an inside job. Of course, as gay people we know that we don't have a lot in the way of external freedom—there is no doubt whatsoever that we have been cast by the "external powers" that be as an illegitimate child of civilization.

It was the activism of those who lived before me that gave me a platform to freedom. Nevertheless, only by being born into a world where it was equally assumed and accepted that I could be gay instead of straight and given all of the same external rights and acceptance could I have avoided being faced with a serious personal challenge. And if I had not accepted this challenge myself, the activism and the hard-won external freedoms would have been wasted on me, as they sit unutilized by an untold number of gay men in the world today.

This is because societal legitimacy is only a platform—the choices that a person makes in his own internal journey to freedom are ultimately the only choices that matter, and they determine how free that person truly is.

At this point in time it is easy to look out on the forces of gay activism in the world to create enclaves of legitimacy to believe that we are on the brink. Indeed fighting for equal external opportunity is our imperative, and it is as noble as the fight for freedom for women, people of African descent, poor people, or any subjugated group anywhere in the world.

But no law can ever make you valid, nor can it make you invalid, because nothing external can change your divine, perfect nature. Only your own belief in homophobia can make you feel invalid, and only your own personal sense of your inherent validity can give you the freedom from oppression that you seek.

External Legitimacy Cannot Heal You

Just as seeking happiness in someone else is a nonstarter, seeking legitimacy from a person or group or society can never deliver on its promise. Even at its very best—say in the way heterosexuals are thought of in this world—external legitimacy can easily turn into enslavement and numbness. If external legitimacy were the answer, heterosexuals would be in heaven. Take a look at the world and you will see that they are far from heaven indeed.

In the case of sexuality, with no challenge to their authenticity, billions of heterosexuals have little or no need to wake up from their unconscious state because the breast of external acceptance is never pulled away. But out gay men tend to be much more conscious and aware of sex and gender "rules" because they were compelled by their own nature to reject the breast milk of heterosexual society that was poisonous to them. And it was in rejecting what society imposed on them that they were able to create something consciously on their own that was right for them and that they knew from personal experience was true. And so the poison turned out to be an elixir because it woke gay men up. That poison milk certainly woke me up!

This is the true gift to being gay. In contemporary Western society, the common journey of a young gay man is to wake up in a world that is sick with homophobia, but then he hears the call of another belief system, one that indicates he's perfectly fine, in fact, maybe even better than fine: maybe he's more fabulous, more creative, more interesting, better looking, you name it. So at first he believes he's inferior, then he is led to believe that he's fine, and maybe he's even superior.

Certainly this was my journey. But as you know my need to feel validated by gay society came from the unconscious beliefs I still held that I was invalid because I was gay. And thus whereas there was once a defeated victim of homophobia, there was now a person struggling with an internal war because both images of myself still existed in my head.

As with me, this war is only real to those for whom the battle inside is still being waged. Take a look at activists for any group. Many activists are riddled with fear, which comes out in the form of anger, self-righteousness, agitation, conflict and anxiety. Being on the "right" side of things does not necessarily mean you are enlightened, but it can be a powerful crutch for everyone in the world who wants to feel that they are in the light but who do not want to face their own demons. In this unconscious and projecting state of living, they feel that if they do not defeat an external evil, evil will win.

The problem is that those who are dominantly on the dark side, such as anti-gay groups, feel exactly the same. This is how the mythology of *Star Wars* got it so right—you can be in the light, but if you are still trying to defeat darkness in others, it means that darkness is still in you, and the longer you continue, the stronger it becomes. Being riddled with fear and trying to exterminate an external "evil" are the hallmarks of darkness and unconscious living. So it is your darkness with which you must do battle, because it is only your own darkness that you can defeat. *That* is the hallmark of a conscious person, and that is the attitude a conscious gay person has about homophobia, because homophobia is just another expression of darkness.

Conscious activists are entirely different creatures. They are at rest in the truth because they have realized it themselves. They do not seek from others what they already have, which is a complete sense of validity. They do not create conflict, nor do they confuse themselves with their cause. Instead, coming from a place of peace and awareness, they spread peace and awareness. And this is the mark of the only kind of truly effective activist there is—one who does not expect others to make them right. They know truth, and the truth is that evil does not exist for you if it does not exist in you.

This internal sense of legitimacy is the reason there are always dramatic exceptions to whatever rules prevail about people. Rupert Everett and Ellen DeGeneres have both sacrificed what they thought they could "get" from pretending to be straight for what they could do by being who they are. And George Michael has written beautiful, insightful and sophisticated pop music about his own gay experiences despite music industry dogma that nothing "gay" would sell.

In each case the same thing can be seen, which is an absence of a bias against themselves. This manifests the transmutation of what the environmental activist Jane Goodall calls "just me-ism"—which is the paralysis you feel when you look out into the world and think that the problems are too big for you to do anything about—into authentic power, which is what Mahatma Gandhi meant when he said, "You must be the change you want to see in the world."

To Eradicate Homophobia, Discover Its True Nature

When it comes to realizing truth as it relates to homophobia, you must see homophobia for what it is: it is a fear, and fear comes from the ego, which is the human's belief that he or she is alone and cut off from the All. Therefore like fear and ego, homophobia is an illusion. That is the truth. If you believe in homophobia, you project it onto other people and then think that you must resist homophobes. But if you eradicate evil in yourself, in this case manifested as homophobia, it will be seen for what it truly is, an illusion, and it will then disappear.

For those who think that I am not being "realistic" by suggesting that renouncing homophobia is the way to defeat it, I would say this: the most effective way to disempower anything is to realize it does not exist. In believing that homophobia does exist, you empower it. And why in the world would you want to empower something that is against you? For ideas such as racism or homophobia or prejudice of any sort, the ideas are real *only to those who believe them.* Nazis, white supremacists, and ethnic cleansers completely believe their utterly fictional racist mythology. Thus it is real to them because they created it and they see the "reality" of it everywhere they look. For those of us who do not believe it, it is not real: it is seen for what it is, which is an insane illusion.

Homophobia is no different. If you believe in its existence, it reveals that part of you believes it is true. How can you stamp out an external enemy when it has taken hold of your own mind? The imperative then is to clean it from your own mind, thereby, removing your contribution to homophobia's "reality." That is all you can ever do for the world, which is to be the change you want to see.

So when you feel anger or fear or pain or the need to be right when it comes to homophobia, find where it is hiding in you, dispel the illusion and, by virtue of that act, renounce it altogether.

Two friends of mine who were dating each other went out to

eat one time. The one who had been to the restaurant before told the other one that the place was "very straight" and that they shouldn't hold hands because it would make other people uncomfortable. The innocent one looked around and felt no fear and saw no indication of this, but he decided to take his boyfriend's word on faith, thinking, well, maybe it would cause a fuss. That minute, a drag queen came in with a big gay entourage and was welcomed with great enthusiasm by the host who knew the group well. The two both got a big laugh over it. This is no doubt a very benign example, but the point is that one of them projected homophobia and saw it everywhere; the other didn't and he experienced no bias against himself until his boyfriend planted it there. This is how we contribute to homophobia—it uses us as its tool to stay real.

How to Use Homophobia as a Learning Tool

As with all challenges to authenticity, homophobia's effect on my life isn't what my inner lion wants, but it is what I as a whole, conscious being need because it exposes in me an excuse to reject my perfection and deny myself love and happiness. That's all homophobia is anyway to gay people who believe in it—an *excuse*, among many others, to hate themselves. And as with every other element of our journey, we get exactly what we are ready for. Homophobia and legitimacy are no different from any of the other forces we have to deal with—it isn't that they are "wrong" or "right," but that they are here for us to grow from.

This does not mean activism is wrong or a dead end. It also doesn't mean that you put your tail between your legs and walk away because they are right about you. What it means is that the only real activism is internal—because effective activism is simply an expression of your internal light. Women and minorities pretty much have no choice when it comes to acknowledging what role they play. Gays, on the other hand, have a choice.

This choice makes the challenge considerably greater, but it also makes the rewards just as grand. The very act of questioning is the act of waking up. It is looking around the dream and asking, "Is this a dream?" If the dream has conformed to you, you will have no need to question it. But the dream rarely conforms to gay people, and thus we are given a spiritual gift . . . if we choose to take it.

In Western society today droves and droves of gay men are choosing to take this gift, which is wonderful news. But what frequently happens is that they wake up just enough to switch the dream around to a gay one, then they go right back to sleep. Meanwhile they are still victimized by the old dream, for the dream of external illegitimacy creates the need for the dream of external legitimacy. And then they become victimized by the new dream, too, which insists they march to the gay drum, even if it is straight off a cliff.

Which dream is true—the one that says we are hideous, shadowy, pathetic, weak, worthless pedophiles, or the one that says we are gorgeous, buff, masculine, Gucci-wearing, sophisticated hunks? Maybe neither. Only a look deep inside can release you from what seems to be an outside struggle but which is, in fact, your own struggle to discern what is real and what is not.

Whose reality do you believe? How about Egypt, where you go to prison if you're gay? Or what about Amsterdam, where you can get married if you're gay? If you pick any of them you're in trouble, because as soon as you travel your sense of your legitimacy changes. If you pick none of them but instead rely on your own, then you're truly legitimate no matter what any magistrate, mullah, minister or mayor has to say. This is why my friend Daryl feels free to be openly gay wherever he is, but his boyfriend, Erik, insists the world is too dangerous to be openly gay anywhere except for the gayest of gay surroundings, and even there he's on shaky ground because you never know who will see you. The only difference between them is that Daryl listens to his own heart, while Erik is still plugged in to the program.

Do Your Part to End Homophobia's Reign by Eradicating It in Yourself

If you want to be legitimate and if you want to make a world in which everyone is liberated from homophobia, the only real thing you can do is rid yourself of it. This means constant questioning of your "reality"—endless vigilance to make sure you have not gone back to sleep into a dream where gay men have enough freedoms to party, to fuck and to be fabulous and that's all you need to know.

Remember that what you judge and criticize the most is what you know to be a part of yourself that you do not want to accept. Any time you are upset by a homophobic assertion of any kind or an assault on your validity from a person or a group, it is simply your own pain being exposed. And more insidiously, any negative feelings you have about gay men—they're so fucked up, they're addicted to drugs, they're too feminine, they're a bunch of clones—is you doing the persecuting because you yourself are one of homophobia's foot soldiers. And it is how you truly feel about yourself.

Any time you stop criticizing someone else for their homophobia and you dig down deep to hear your own inner voices say that *they are right about you,* you have taken the opportunity to clean yourself up, become more conscious, and make your flame brighter. Heal yourself of the poison that says you are imperfect and wrong and less and not as good because you are gay, and you have dissolved homophobia for yourself forever and taken away the power you were giving to its "reality" in the world. The beautiful thing is that when you do, you will then be given opportunities to light the flame for others. That's the way Spirit or Consciousness or God or whatever you want to call it works.

You do not need a national platform. I was first introduced to my thirteen-year-old "little brother" Greg through Big Brothers Big Sisters when I was thirty. When I first met him he regularly said "faggot" in response to gay characters in movies or gay men he saw in my neighborhood. And when I first heard him say it, I found myself quite angry. All it took to shake me up were the comments of a thirteen-year-old. And I was a big, fabulous gay man in Manhattan!

So I looked deep inside and found that part of me was afraid he was right. It took months before I was clean enough that he could say "faggot," and I wasn't upset in the least. Then I was able to see what was going on clearly: he'd absorbed some bad ideas from the culture, it had nothing to do with me, and I could now help counteract it by introducing him to the truth, but without need for him to agree.

That was when the right thing to say started to come to me, which is to say, I asked the Universe to guide me and it did. When he would say something derogatory, I started off by suggesting that the word "faggot" is no different than the "n" word (Greg is black), and would he like it if someone used that word around him? The next time he said it I suggested that he undoubtedly knows people who are gay, only he doesn't know they are gay, and that every time he says it he is hurting them like he would be hurt with the "n" word. Later on I added that for all he knew *I* was gay. And each time I said anything I felt no anger nor a need to be right—quite the opposite; I was probably as gentle as I'd ever been in my life.

A year into our relationship I was invited to a family event, and I decided to bring a date in order to finally get it across to Greg that I was indeed gay. My date, Earl, and I were sitting at a table full of Greg's male teenage cousins when one of them copped on that Earl and I looked like we were dating. Earl said that we indeed were, and at that moment I wouldn't have been surprised if a tumbleweed had gone rolling across the table it was so still. Then suddenly Greg chimed in, "I knew it all along!" like he was trying to be cool! Can you imagine? And suddenly we were back to normality, with all his cousins begging me to take them on a group trip to Manhattan. And in one fell swoop six black teenage boys from Queens and the Bronx learned that it is normal and right to be gay. All it took to have that effect was one gay individual who felt that way, too. Just one.

This is the power to change the world that each of us possesses. And I have begun to access this power, because I'm not waiting around for a president or a pope or a parent or anyone else to tell me I exist. I know I exist. And it is the very challenges to my existence that have brought me to realization of truth about myself and homophobia. The number one truth about homophobia is this: at its deepest core it is a fear and hatred of the feminine in ourselves, which is really a fear and hatred of the power of creation, and that is a fear and hatred of the one, unified force of love, intelligence and creation from which we all come and are an inherent part of, but which we have rejected.

Homophobia is simply the expression of that rejection.

Jane Goodall talked about how "just me-ism" is paralyzing and an illusion, and this is exactly what I mean. You can look around the world and be paralyzed by the war against gay people and think there is nothing you can do. Or you might think that screaming at people will do the job. What does the job is lighting that flame in yourself by casting away your own darkness. If every single gay person in the world did it, homophobia as an external institution and a powerful force would collapse instantaneously because it cannot survive without our support. So how can you make that happen? Light your flame.

Who Are You?

Know thyself.

—The Delphic Oracle

M any people, regardless of their beliefs, eventually turn to "spirituality" or "self-help" because they want to be happy. And simply wanting to feel better—not finding God or spirituality or what is referred to in classical philosophy as "the Self"—might very well be why you were drawn to this book.

But there is one desire that goes even deeper than the desire to be happy and to feel good that all people know in their core because they were born with it and they live with it every second of every day. This desire haunts secularists, atheists and fundamentalists alike. Yet this particular desire is the backstory of our motivations even before the desire to be happy. This backstory of all backstories is literally the essence of the human condition, and it expresses itself in a question we are all born with and can never shake no matter how hard we try. And the question is, "Who am I?"

Before we are even born our answers are prepared for us. You are your name, you were born on such and such a date, and these are your parents from whom you came. After we are born, we unconsciously begin to make our own deductions, such as "I am this body," "I am this emotion I'm experiencing," "I am this name," and "I am this need that I have."

As we grow older and soak in more ideas from the culture and create ideas that indicate what is right and good about us and what is wrong or missing in us, we develop an increasingly complex and sophisticated answer to this question. We begin to have literally hundreds of mostly unconscious answers to the question and they are often in a state of extreme flux, such as "I am what I own," "I am my political party," "I am my successes," "I am my appearance," "I am my failures," "I am crazy," "I am a slut," "I am no good," "I am my gender," "I am brilliant," "I am twenty," "I am thirty," "I am my religion," "I am my community," "I am my race," and on and on and on.

And as soon as you find there are differences in sexual preferences you begin to identify with those as well, which is why many gay men will answer "I am straight" at one point in their life, and then "I am gay" at another.

Underneath it all is the battle between your conflicting ideas about yourself in the form of your various self-images, not to mention all your ideas about the world, because you think you are those as well.

Even deeper than that is a feeling that we *are* our pain because it is the only thing that seems to follow us everywhere we go, and so it becomes our unconscious foundation of reality and identification. This is, as it says in *A Course in Miracles,* the ego's false sense of security—by making you believe that you can't escape from pain the ego ensures its existence. After all, if you believe that you are pain and you successfully release it then you no longer exist. So in order to not disappear, you unconsciously choose to believe, "I am pain."

The Pressing Nature of the Question

The endless clinging to these conflicting and often horrible answers reveals the pressing nature of the question. As we get older and we watch various pillars of our identity crash—I no longer am what I looked like, I no longer am the relationship I was in, I no longer am the career I once had—we seek out new ones to identify with and have faith in. But no matter what the pillar nor how long it has stood, we still feel terrified about what is going to happen to us when that pillar collapses and turns to dust. Naturally we deduce that we need to renew our efforts in building up our pillars or find newer and bigger ones, hence why some people become addicted to plastic surgery to maintain their physical image, while others become obsessed with maintaining the power of their religion or political party. It's all about keeping themselves alive by keeping their self-images alive.

But if we live long enough to get old, we've watched enough of our pillars crash to feel substantially *diminished*. At thirty-five I've already experienced this—it has taken me years to get over the sense that I am less now that I am no longer a twenty-eight-year-old shirtless bartender in Chelsea high on the spotlight. And though that's small potatoes, it still hurt to give up because it was a self-image that I loved and I desperately wanted to be.

As everything we ever reach for dissolves before our eyes, we begin to ask on a very deep level, "What or who is left?" This *need* for security, for something that is permanent and unbreakable and immortal, is so massive a need that, as unwilling as we are to truly address the question, we are willing to numb ourselves of its eternal nagging.

People often turn to religion for a quick answer—a particular God created them, and they will go to heaven if they believe in Him—and the question is answered for them. Others, who are skeptical of religion, will turn to science to answer the question—they came from the big bang, and they are made up of hydrogen and carbon atoms—and so they choose not only to believe in nothing, they *believe* in Nothing.

Meanwhile, each group is still clinging—to their family names, to their bodies, to their jobs, to their reputations, to their possessions, to their ideas, to their fears, to their political parties—and the acid test is that they feel monumentally threatened when anything they identify with is challenged.

All of these crazy reactions, which are at the bottom of

religious, political, social and familial wars, come from the unquenchable thirst to know, "Who am I?" The belief that we are separate and on our own in a brutal cosmos is the fear-based answer to the question, and it is the life experience of both believers in God and believers in Nothing, for belief is not the answer. Realization is.

How to Use Your Own Mind to Figure Out Who You Really Are

I have already passed on the skills to help you see that you are not your reactions, your character, your sexual tastes, your fears, your boyfriend, your hopes, your beliefs, your addictions, or anything else that is blocking your ability to experience awareness and to feel happy. But now we come to the real point of all of this work, which is to help you answer the question, "Who am I?"

The essential lesson you have been taught so far is the power of observation. What do you see when you observe? You witness different emotions; you see changes everywhere; you observe results from different intentions and reactions. The essential thing you observe, though, is *change*. Everything you are learning to observe is born, develops, decays, then dies. Everything, including reactions and thoughts and beliefs, come into being and then leave. Religion and science are both subject to the force of birth, decay and death as well. Even the mighty sun will one day collapse in on itself and blow itself and the solar system to bits. Nothing, and I mean absolutely nothing in the physical universe, is permanent, except for change.

This is the first lesson of observation because you learn it applies to everything you thought was "you," which is why your old answers made you feel so fragile. Then you see from the standpoint of the observer that all those things come and go, but the one doing the observing stays still. And now you begin to learn that if you identify and attach with anything you can observe—if on some level you think it *is* you—you will suffer, because one minute it will be there, then it will not. Except for the pain that you endlessly create—that somehow seems eternal.

But where do we go from here? Where is the answer? No need to panic, because it's right here, though it's not anything you can observe. That's because it, or rather you, *are* the observer. You *are* the entity that is witnessing all of this—it is the you behind the you at ten, twenty, forty, fifty. It is the one experiencing pain and pleasure, sadness and laughter, luck and misfortune, knowledge and ignorance, sex and hunger, on and on. It is the you at the center of a gigantic tornado you call your life.

The tricky thing is that the observer can't be observed. Up until now you might have only been aware of what you could observe, which is why that was all you had to go on when it came to figuring out who you are. But while the observer cannot be seen, it can be identified with, and this is the answer you seek because it is the condition you seek, for it is unshakeable. You want to feel secure? Then feel your own nature.

How do you go about identifying with the observer instead of what you can observe? You do so by no longer identifying with what you are not. In other words, I can't tell you that you are God or Consciousness or Knowledge or the All and have it mean anything real to you. These are just words on a page— symbols, ideas, directions. *What you have to do is remove everything you are not in order to realize what you are.*

How Realizing Your True Nature Changes the Way You See the Universe

When you find the will to let go of the idea that you are any of your observations—including the things you might really treasure like your money or your talent or your looks or your reputation—you find yourself considerably less shaken by change or threatened in any way. Slowly your need to be right diminishes; your need to impress people becomes less valuable to you; your clinging to people or places that you thought you couldn't do without slowly gets released. The winds of change blow and you feel steady. Why is this? Because in not believing you are any of these things that you observe and that are subject to change you realize through sheer experience you are that which is not subject to change, the witness to all of this.

This is what is meant by self-realization: it is literally realizing your true self. And it *is* your purpose for being here on this Earth, though again this is meaningless coming from me—it will only have meaning when you realize it yourself. That is the true meaning behind, "To thine own self be true." Shakespeare was both a humanist and a philosopher, and by the "self" he meant every aspect of the self, from the ego to the Divine. It's not just about being true to the self on Earth that you experience. That's only the first step, and acknowledging that the self you experience on Earth is gay is a big one. The next step is being true to the self that does the experiencing, including the experience of your sexuality. That's how in your journey toward self-knowledge you go from "I am not gay," to "I am gay," to "*I am not gay*," but with a whole different meaning—and it isn't "ex-gay" because straight people aren't straight either!

What are the qualities to this witness, to your true self? You have to see for yourself. I can feel that it, or rather *me*, is utterly still, forever in the present and never changes in any way. And so, deep inside, I find exactly what I have been searching for outside of myself in the form of men or approval or reputation or any of those things I used to cherish so much.

Through lifting these veils and identifying with the observer, you begin to see the true nature of the universe and the true nature of everyone you know and meet because your true nature and everyone else's true nature and every thing are one and the same. You not only become receptive to the fact that everything exists in relationship to everything else (something the secular and religious worlds are coming to terms with now via the science of quantum physics—that everything on the Earth and in the cosmos is a single part of one whole), you begin to *see and feel* oneness.

This sense of oneness is a bit like a pool of water that you wade in wherever you go so that it's always with you. As you continue to work on your journey, the threshold gets higher. At one point it was only around your ankles, and then you begin to feel it around your legs. Then sometimes grace steps in, and you feel awash in it—which is what happened to me the night I was awash in a tidal wave of consciousness and reborn while walking home from my friend Christian's that rainy April night. I felt unbelievably awake, and I saw beauty and perfection in everything and everyone I laid my eyes on. My perception was so intense and vivid that everything brought me joy—everything was knowledge, light and love wrapped up in one. Even the couches in the furniture store were radiating beautiful meaning.

My mind was no longer clouded by illusion as the entire arc of my own life was presented to me. In a flash I could see that I had believed that every person was born with a certain amount of goods to work with–looks, love, intelligence, talent, and so on–which I visualized as a small, white paper bag. I had spent my whole life afraid to put my hand all the way in the bag out of fear that I'd find out I had been screwed over. That was the true source of all the bitterness and jealousy I'd ever felt. In the vision I put my hand all the way in and saw that my gift bag was fuller than I could ever have imagined.

But then, unexpectedly, my hand burst through the bottom of the bag, my fist opened up on the other side and, in a singular moment of profound realization, I knew that I wasn't my gift bag, and I knew I wasn't my pain in its various forms. *I* was infinite; *I* was knowledge; *I* was light; *I* was love. The reason I was seeing it everywhere was because I had always seen the world as I am, the only difference was at this moment I was realizing my true identity.

It is in this new state of awareness that you begin to get the ridiculousness of the idea of separation–after all, even in the physical cosmos everything is made up of the same stuff and nothing can exist on its own. As Carl Sagan pointed out, your body is made of "star stuff." Believing that you are separate from everything else is like your liver declaring independence. It is simply ludicrous. But if your liver did try to be separate, it would have the same consequences on the body that our belief in separation is having on each other and on the Earth–disaster and death.

Realizing there is no separation is also how your ability to be violent disappears. Your belief that someone else is "bad" goes away, and your disrespect for life transmutes into awe and reverence because you see one and the same self in everything and everything in yourself. This is when "gay and straight," "good and bad," "Republican and Democrat," "old and young," and "right and wrong" slowly dissolve. You see life as one single force, and every expression of life that you see is simply a mirror of the life that you are. The most powerful illusions of the universe are inch by inch dispelled. Suddenly you find yourself on a different plane of existence entirely, though you're standing on the same damn spot. This has been true for me. I still live on 8th and 21st in Chelsea, yet I now live in a fundamentally different universe.

The nature of the cosmos that begins to be revealed to you is one of *giving.* As someone said once, in all these years the Sun has never looked at the Earth and said, "You owe me." Giving is what the universe does. Giving is what life and love is. Because you are no longer identified with your fear and your need to get, you begin to give freely and see that you are being given to freely as well. The universe turns from something you had believed was constantly taking from you to something that is forever giving to you. And because you, too, are the universe, giving is naturally the thing to do.

You will also discover something awesomely powerful about the observer, which is that it lives in the eternal present. It is always here, and it is always now. The observer, which is to say you, is never off reliving a past event or fretting over an imagined future one. In fact you see that all there is is the present, and it is all that will ever be. And in the present nothing that causes you pain—fear, anxiety, addiction, desperation, or even hope, because without fear you don't need it—can exist. Up in a poof of awareness goes all that suffering that you thought was just the nature of life and the only eternal thing you knew. And what an unbelievable relief and surprise that is. Your worst fears about yourself are not true. *Your worst fears about life are not true.*

This is especially potent because it releases you from self-judgment and criticism, for after all you are *none* of the things you can observe, including your fears and destructive habits. You created all that pain (including guilt and judgment over the pain), you can uncreate it, and now it's gone.

And the big big thing you will see is the insanity of the idea of a brutal, meaningless, mindless cosmos, or the idea that there is a God, but "He" is hateful and you are separate from "Him." Insanity is chaos of the mind, and when in a state of chaos, that is what you see. Insanity doesn't really exist, but you can create it and believe in it so that it's true to you. Sanity, on the other hand, is the natural order of the mind that is simply allowed to be, and in that state you see order and meaning everywhere. You see a picture of a galaxy or a snowflake or Saturn, and you see the most magnificent mind there ever was behind it all. And what is on this mind is truly grand—the very essence of fun, beauty, grandeur, elegance, innocence, love, wisdom, complexity, infinity and simplicity. It *is* intelligence, joy and knowledge. It is consciousness itself. And it is you. Look upon God and see yourself.

It is also a profoundly flamboyant mind, as one look at a waterfall, a supernova or an impossibly complex and ordered ice crystal reveals. My neighbor Lori's dog, Ronin, doesn't do anything that isn't outrageously flamboyant—even the way he is built with almond eyes, a white chest, and a curly caramel tail couldn't have been created except by the most unabashedly flamboyant designer who would, no doubt, be assumed gay if he were a man. When my devoted cat, Moo, is in the mood for love her long, white whiskers curve down and out, framing her mouth in a display so luxurious and flamboyant that it puts Liberace to shame. Sagi's dog, Neo, spends his whole life celebrating existence and demonstrates it by wagging his whole body. And to think all that homophobia in the world that is so opposed to flamboyance is really an opposition to God itself. Realizing that homophobia is in fact God-phobia is quite a leap in understanding its nature, wouldn't you say? And this is the benefit of realization.

As you continue on this path you will begin to see symmetry and perfection everywhere, including in events you initially think are "bad." Everywhere you look you see love and knowledge, for both rain down from the heavens and are radiated out of the eyes of every living creature you see. You see knowledge and consciousness and the essence of the one ultimate being in everything there is. How in the world would my palm tree, which knows how to push out grand fans of bright olive green that can turn sunlight into energy, be able to to do what it does without knowledge and consciousness? Are you saying it performs the impossible because it's dumb? You will see all living organisms' true nature as knowledge and consciousness because you will know your own.

In that moment you will recognize that all true knowledge is self-knowledge, because in knowing yourself, you know everything that is true and everything that is real. You will see that other people, too, aren't their ideas—even if they don't see this. And what better help could you be to the person suffering from bad ideas than to be a mirror to reflect their real self? This is The Answer to peace on Earth—instead of conflict you perpetuate love.

You will finally accept that denying a creator when presented not only with your own existence but also an infinitely complex, conscious and beautiful universe is more insane than denying the creator of a simple oil painting—yet you would certainly think it insane to believe an oil painting came from nowhere. And who is this creator? It is you.

So what was insane becomes sane, and vice versa. And you make the decidedly logical decision to stick with what you now know and feel from personal experience to be sanity. Other people can continue to choose what you now realize is insanity, but your choice to be sane is yours and you've made it. You've become sane by learning who you truly are.

**8**

Change Is Possible

I'm living my life like it's golden.

—Jill Scott

I have changed. Or rather, the way I experience my life has changed, and as a result the personality I experience as Chris has changed a lot, too.

Before, I was constantly running from fear and pain—they were my lens, my nemesis, and my utterly unquestioned reality. These days it's quite a different story. Of course, after having spent decades building that character it is still functioning in my mind. The difference is that whereas before it reigned unquestioned as my reality, it is now seen for the dream that it is, and in the process it is dissolving.

Unlike the old personalities that had to be constructed, my new reality has only to be revealed, which indicates to me that this is my natural state of being. I now focus on the real, unseen meaning behind events rather than the superficial, illusory, fear-based meaning that used to be my reality. And this is as big a change as can occur—in fact it is the only real change there is; everything else is simply a moving around of the illusion.

Of course, there are lots of people out there who insist that, "People don't change." "Same shit, different day!" they say because they carry their own shit everywhere they go. This is the force you will be up against as you begin to give in to happiness. Others do not want you to change because it is a threat to their choice not to. I used to believe that I could never come out of the closet or love myself because I was gay. Now I am out to the entire world, and not only do I love myself, I am on the path to realizing that I *am* love. I used to be depressed; now I'm not. I used to be addicted; now I'm considerably less addicted to my habitual patterns. I used to be terrified; now I'm not. So what changed? I changed. That's all I need to know.

Changing is a matter of making the single change to let go of your ego's idea of yourself, whether it's a closeted gay man or

a fabulous gay man or a straight-acting gay man or a gay victim, whatever. It means giving up everything you have built to
deny who you are. It means facing that gigantic black hole
inside of yourself that you turned your back on—and being
brave enough to turn around and look straight into its heart.

You will find the motivation to change when you remove
your cover-ups, feel the pain that is rotting away at your being,
decide you *do not want to feel like that anymore,* and decide, in
fact, that you'll do anything to not feel like that anymore.

Changing Requires Bravery

I'm not saying you don't have to be brave. My good friend
Jose realized in the middle of a party in Miami how he had been
replicating the same experience for a dozen years: getting high,
picking up a guy, crashing, and doing it all over again, and he
was now forty. In that one moment he did not judge himself or
his friends, but he did say, I've done this enough, and I'm no
longer getting anything out of it. He then hopped on a plane and
came back to New York. Changing his habits, going through
withdrawal, facing the fear and judgment from his friends who
are taking his changes personally, and letting his reality evolve
into something new has not been easy. But he's on his way, and
realizing his potential to re-create his reality has given him so
much enthusiasm that, so different from the strung-out and
upset Jose I used to know, almost every time I see him now he
tells me how *powerful* he feels.

Like Jose, discovering that the way out is, in fact, the way *in* will
be a big, big change for you. In searching inside for my answers
I have discovered things I simply never considered or even imagined. Elements of my life that seemed utterly rigid are breaking

apart like giant icebergs melting in the sun. I'll look in the mirror and catch myself starting to belittle myself as I have done for decades, and I'll stop myself right there. Are you kidding? I don't have to do that anymore. *I do not have to do that anymore.* I catch myself starting to feel embarrassed to be gay in front of the straight guys on the basketball court, and I think, no, there is nothing to be embarrassed about. I am gay, and I am perfect.

As a result I can enjoy my life. At times I feel like the R&B poet-singer Jill Scott sings: "I'm living my life like it's golden." When you begin to feel this way you will then be given glimpses of what life is like in the light, like the big one I had that I consider my moment of rebirth. And you will then be changed forever.

Yet and still, surrendering to happiness is difficult, which raises the question, what is so wrong with infinite bliss that I continue to work to deny it even though it is being offered? Well, the fact is that other things are still more important to me, and as long as they are, that's what I'll have. *A Course in Miracles* says that "from what you want, God does not save you," and that is the point. If it's pain and future and past that I want—if getting to the gym is more important than loving myself—that's what I'll get. And there's nothing wrong with it because that is how I'm learning. As much as I want to allow in the bliss that is being offered, I'll have it. You can see I still have a long way to go on my path, but now I know that I am on one, and I know which one it is.

Everything happens on its own timetable. The shedding of a snake's skin cannot be rushed—it happens when it happens. But it's not about waiting to be enlightened and waiting to change in order to be happy—it's about loving and accepting yourself right now. That is enlightenment.

Trust and see that realization can make the impossible happen and you will experience a change. As you ascend, being, knowing and having begin to merge into a single dynamic, one unified force within you. This is a condition that toddlers like my nephew, Rhett, and my neighbor Lori's baby, Cate, know so well, and that we can return to once we make the necessary changes.

Higher Awareness Is Not a Bunch of Bullshit

The very idea of a place of awareness that is "higher" is anathema to a lot of people—it's a bunch of crap, it's all fake, it's mumbo-jumbo, it's just another cult. Yet it is such an integral part of life that we know. How is it that you can at one time of your life exist in a womb and not even know where you are or that you exist, and later know indisputably that you exist in a measureless cosmos with billions of people, and then turn around and deny different levels of consciousness? The evidence of different states of consciousness is all around us and takes place throughout our own lifetimes—it takes a feat of profound arrogance to deny that there is any state beyond what you know now, and of profound defiance to not want to recognize that this higher state is inside of you.

In other words, change is possible though you, your true self, will not change. Only your experience of your life will change as you connect with your true self. Trust that your experience can and will change. The universe is endlessly young, forever new each minute. So are you. It's only the idea that it's still the same stuff all over again that makes you experience life that way. But if you hold those old outcomes in mind, let them go, and step back into your reality open and certain that something new will unfold, it truly will. That is when you will discover that you are a creator with infinite possibilities. Wake up in the morning, then wake up again and again and again throughout the day, and you will see serious changes. You will no longer be trapped.

The idea that gay culture cannot change stems from our own individual lies to ourselves that *we* cannot change. But if you as an individual make the choice to change, you will do your part to help gay society transform from the dynamic of pain and using each other that we have become so numb to, to a frequency of love and giving to one another that will bring about a true gay heaven. And in doing this you will help change the world. It can happen—it can totally happen, but only if you make this change yourself.

In high school I had a dark fascination with my friend Mary Margaret's rabbit, who lived in a cage in their garage and literally never came out or saw the sun. I couldn't believe he existed like that, so one beautiful spring day I took the cage out into the backyard, opened it up, and eagerly waited for him to come out and play and be free. But he didn't. So I then tipped the cage over, and he had no choice but to slip out onto the grass. But as soon as the cage was flat again he scurried back in. Feeling defeated, I eventually gave up, shut the door to the cage and sadly returned him to the dark garage.

I could never comprehend why he would choose to live like that, that is, until decades later when I realized that I was him, that I had chosen pain over freedom because I was too afraid of change. But I don't want to be him anymore, and so I choose to run toward freedom regardless of how afraid I might be. And that was his gift to me.

This change *is* the journey. Everyone on the planet has the same journey before them, which is to realize who we truly are, and in doing so release ourselves from our cages and find the freedom, the happiness, the acceptance and the perfection that has been waiting for us all along. The journey begins with "Who am I?" and ends when you have fully realized the only answer there is.

Now, go seek your answer.

About the Author

Christopher Lee Nutter is a freelance journalist who has written for *The Village Voice*, *Details* magazine, *The Advocate*, *The New York Times*, *Vibe*, *The Gay and Lesbian Review Worldwide* and others. He lives in New York City.

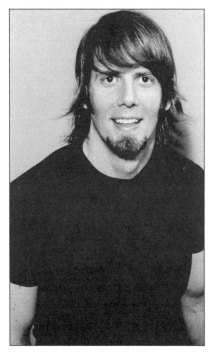

Author photo by Atila Marquez

Visit his Web site at: *www.christopherleenutter.com.*

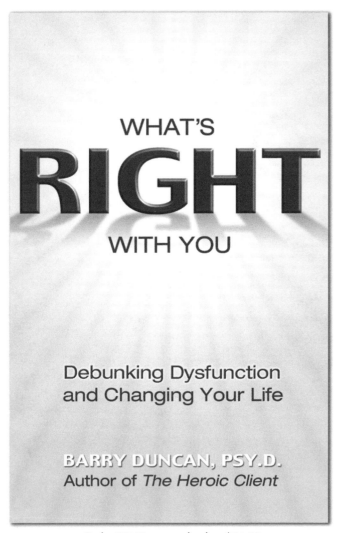

WHAT'S RIGHT WITH YOU

Debunking Dysfunction and Changing Your Life

BARRY DUNCAN, PSY.D.
Author of *The Heroic Client*

Code #2548 • paperback • $14.95

Tap into your inner resilience and change your life in 6 dynamic and easy-to-follow steps!

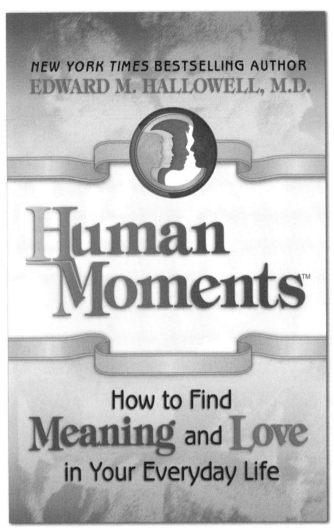

NEW YORK TIMES BESTSELLING AUTHOR
EDWARD M. HALLOWELL, M.D.

Human Moments™

How to Find
Meaning and Love
in Your Everyday Life

Code #9101 • paperback • $12.95

Discover today how to live the rewarding and meaningful life you've always dreamed. Let renowned psychiatrist and bestselling author Edward M. Hallowell teach you the secret in this unique and provocative book.

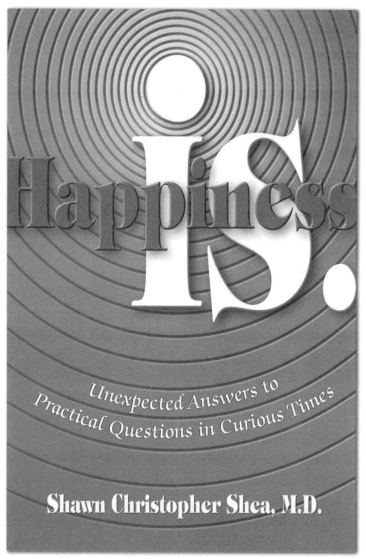

Happiness is.

Unexpected Answers to Practical Questions in Curious Times

Shawn Christopher Shea, M.D.

Code #0669 • hardcover • $19.95

Written with elegance, wit and a disarming playfulness, Dr. Shea provides invaluable tools for finding your own unique answers to the puzzle of happiness.
